OPCS Surveys of Psychiatric
Morbidity in Great Britain

Report 4

# The prevalence of psychiatric morbidity among adults living in institutions

Howard Meltzer

Baljit Gill

Mark Petticrew

Kerstin Hinds

London: HMSO

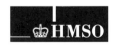

Published by HMSO and available from:

**HMSO Publications Centre**
(Mail, fax and telephone orders only)
PO Box 276, London SW8 5DT
Telephone orders 0171 873 9090
General enquiries 0171 873 0011
(queuing system in operation for both numbers)
Fax orders 0171 873 8200

**HMSO Bookshops**
49 High Holborn, London WC1V 6HB
(counter service only)
0171 873 0011  Fax 0171 831 1326
68–69 Bull Street, Birmingham B4 6AD
0121 236 9696   Fax 0121 236 9699
33 Wine Street, Bristol BS1 2BQ
0117 9264306  Fax 0117 9294515
9–21 Princess Street, Manchester M60 8AS
0161 834 7201  Fax 0161 833 0634
16 Arthur Street, Belfast BT1 4GD
01232 238451  Fax 01232 235401
71 Lothian Road, Edinburgh EH3 9AZ
0131 228 4181  Fax 0131 229 2734
The HMSO Oriel Bookshop
The Friary, Cardiff CF1 4AA
01222 395548  Fax 01222 384347

**HMSO's Accredited Agents**
(see Yellow Pages)

*and through good booksellers*

# Authors' acknowledgements

We would like to thank everybody who contributed to the survey and the production of this report. Administrators, medical, nursing and support staff in the establishments we visited were of great assistance to the OPCS interviewers not only in organising contact with respondents but helping as proxy informants when subjects could not manage an interview.

We were supported by our specialist colleagues in OPCS who carried out the sampling, fieldwork, coding and editing stages.

The project was steered by a group comprising the following, to whom thanks are due for assistance and specialist advice at various stages of the survey:

Department of Health:
Dr Rachel Jenkins (chair)
Dr Elaine Gadd
Ms Val Roberts
Ms Antonia Roberts

Psychiatric epidemiologists:
Professor Paul Bebbington
Dr Terry Brugha
Professor Glyn Lewis
Dr Mike Farrell
Dr Jacquie de Alarcon

Office of Population Censuses and Surveys:
Ms Jil Matheson
Dr Howard Meltzer
Ms Baljit Gill
Dr Mark Petticrew
Ms Kerstin Hinds

Most importantly, we would like to thank all the participants in the survey for their co-operation.

# Contents

# Notes

*Tables showing percentages*

Row or column percentages may add to 99% or 101% because of rounding.

The varying positions of the percentage signs and bases in the tables denote the presentation of different types of information. Where there is a percentage sign at the head of a column and the *base* at the foot, the whole distribution is presented and the individual percentages add to between 99% and 101%. Where there is no percentage sign in the table and a note above the figures, the figures refer to the proportion of people who had the attribute being discussed, and the complementary proportion, to add to 100%, is not shown in the table.

The following conventions have been used within tables showing percentages:

|   |   |
|---|---|
| - | no cases |
| 0 | values less than 0.5% |

*2 Significant differences*

The *bases* for some sub-groups presented in the tables were small such that the standard errors around estimates for these groups are biased. Confidence intervals which take account of these biased standard errors were calculated and, although they are not presented in the tables, they were used in testing for statistically significant differences.

# List of tables

# List of figures

# Summary

The OPCS Surveys of psychiatric morbidity in Great Britain were commissioned by the Department of Health, the Scottish Home and Health Department and the Welsh Office. They aim to provide up-to-date information about the prevalence of psychiatric problems among adults in Great Britain as well as their associated social disabilities and use of services.

Four separate surveys were carried out from April 1993 to August 1994.

i) 10,000 adults aged 16 to 64 years living in private households (fieldwork: April 1993 - September 1993)

ii) a supplementary sample of 350 people aged 16 to 64 years with psychosis living in private households (fieldwork: October 1993 - December 1993)

iii) 1,200 people aged 16 to 64 years living in institutions specifically catering for people with mental illness (fieldwork: April 1994 - July 1994)

iv) 1,100 homeless people aged 16 to 64 years living in hostels for the homeless or other such institutions. This sample also included people sleeping rough (fieldwork July 1994 - August 1994)

The results of the surveys are being presented in a series of reports of which this is the fourth. This report focuses on the distribution of psychiatric morbidity among residents of institutions. It also describes how the instruments and the analysis of the data used for the private household survey (see Report 1) were adapted for the institutional survey.

Neurotic psychopathology was measured by the Clinical Interview Schedule - Revised (CIS-R).

Information on psychotic psychopathology was obtained from the reports of residents, or proxy informants (doctors, nurses and other professional staff) who were knowledgable about the subjects' circumstances.

The results of the survey are presented in terms of grossed estimates and prevalence rates of psychiatric disorders by different types and characteristics of institutions.

- In 1994, about 33,200 adults, aged 16 to 64, were permanently resident in accommodation which catered for people with mental health problems. About a third of them were in NHS hospitals; the remainder were in private hospitals (7%) or residential care facilities.

- Seventy percent of adults aged 16 to 64 for whom diagnoses were obtained suffered from schizophrenia, delusional and schizo-affective disorders. This represents 23,100 individuals out of a total estimated establishment population of 33,200. Eight per cent of individuals suffered from neurotic, stress-related or somatoform disorders, and 8% suffered from affective disorders.

- The distribution of the disorders differed according to whether the setting was a hospital or residential accommodation. The prevalence of schizophrenia and related disorders was higher in hospitals, where about three-quarters of residents had this mental health problem compared with two thirds of those in residential accommodation. The prevalence of neurotic disorders was however higher among adults living in residential care.

- The prevalence of schizophrenia and related disorders was higher in NHS psychiatric hospitals and NHS General Hospital units than in private hospitals, clinics or nursing homes. The prevalence of affective disorders was higher in the private establishments, where about one in four residents suffered from this mental health problem compared with one in twelve individuals in NHS establishments.

- When the prevalence of mental health problems among those living in residential accommodation was examined, the only disorder to vary in prevalence between the four residential care settings (residential care homes, group homes, hostels, and ordinary housing or recognised lodgings) was neurosis, the prevalence of which was highest in hostels and lowest in ordinary housing/recognised lodgings.

The prevalence of mental health problems also varied according to who managed the establishment. The prevalence of schizophrenia was higher in accommodation run by Health Authorities or Local Authorities than in accommodation run by the private or voluntary/charitable sector. About three-quarters of people in accommodation managed by a HA or LA, compared to two thirds of those in voluntary/charitable accommodation, suffered from this particular mental health problem.

# 1 Background, aims and coverage of the survey

## 1.1 Background

Mental illness was identified as one of the five key areas for action in *The Health of the Nation*, a White Paper published by the Department of Health in July 1992.[1] The main target in this area was to improve significantly the health and social functioning of people with mental illness. To achieve this goal, it is necessary to have good baseline information about mental illness. In 1992, the Department of Health in conjunction with the Scottish Office and the Welsh Office, therefore commissioned OPCS to carry out a survey of psychiatric morbidity.

The OPCS survey is the first nationally representative survey of psychiatric morbidity to be carried out in Great Britain. There are several other sources of information about mental illness but these data are collected for specific purposes and have limited national applicability.[2] *The Health of the Nation, Key Area Handbook* on mental illness states why the available statistics may underestimate the extent of mental illness in the population: [3]

- the failure to recognise some mental illness at community and primary health care level.

- the failure to recognise psychiatric morbidity in general medical and surgical settings.

- insufficient attention given to psychological distress associated with physical diseases, particularly those associated with long term disablement, for both the patient and their carers.

- the substantial effect of mental illness on other morbidity and mortality statistics and the under-reporting of mental illness due to stigma.

Adults aged 16-64 permanently resident in institutions represent a very small proportion of the total population but are likely to be extensive consumers of health, social and voluntary care services. Although there is information about these residents, the survey offered an opportunity to classify them on the same instruments as those used for the private household survey. Indeed, one of the advantages of carrying out a large national survey of psychiatric morbidity among a representative sample of the institutional population as well as the population in private households was that all informants (regardless of where they live) would be asked the same questions in a standardised way and their answers recorded in the same systematic manner.

## 1.2 Aims of the survey

There were five main aims of the survey.

### Prevalence

One of the main reasons for carrying out the survey in institutions was to estimate the prevalence of psychiatric morbidity according to diagnostic category and type of institution among residents aged 16 to 64 years in Great Britain.

### Social disabilities

The survey aimed to identify the nature and extent of social disabilities associated with mental disorders. Social disabilities refer to the limitations in function or restrictions in activities of people within particular environments. The nature of institutions themselves result in both prescriptions and proscriptions for social functioning, covering social support, social networks and leisure activities.

### Service use

The varying use of services and the receipt of care are examined within each type of institutional setting in relation to type of disorder and their associated social disabilities.

### Recent stressful life events

The survey aimed to investigate how major events in the previous six months were related to how people were feeling at the time of the interview.

### Lifestyle indicators

Another principal aim was to investigate the relationship between mental disorders and smoking, drinking and drug use. Although there are restrictions on such behaviour in many institutions, those living in supported accommodation or group homes have fewer restrictions on their lifestyles. As well as looking at tobacco, alcohol, and drug consumption, particular emphasis was put on the extent of alcohol and drug dependency.

## 1.3 Coverage of the survey

### Region

The population which was surveyed comprised adults living in institutions specifically catering for those with mental health problems in Great Britain (excluding the Highlands and Islands).

### Age

The survey focused on the prevalence of psychiatric morbidity among residents aged 16 to 64. Children, defined as those under the age of 16, and adults aged 65 or above were excluded from the survey. This is because surveys of children's psychopathology and of psychiatric morbidity among elderly people would require specialised sampling, interviewing and assessment procedures.

### Type of institution

This report focuses on the results of the survey which sampled residents in hospitals, residential care homes and alternative types of residential accommodation; institutions whose primary purpose was the long term care of people with mental health disorders. Thus, other types of institutions which have people with mental illness among their residents, such as acute, short-stay HNS hospital facilities, are excluded here. Hostels for homeless people were covered in a separate survey in the research programme (See Report 7)

The survey of residents in institutions was carried out as a separate exercise from the private household survey although the aim was to obtain as much comparable information as possible. Institutional surveys require a separate sampling design, a strategy to negotiate access to the establishment and to the residents, and the use of modified questionnaires. (See Chapter 3).

## 1.4 Coverage of the current report

The main purpose of this Report is to present grossed estimates and prevalence rates of psychiatric morbidity among adults aged 16 to 64 living in institutions in Great Britain. In order to interpret these results, it is important to have an understanding of the conceptual approach and methods adopted for this study, and these are described in Chapters 2 and 3.

Characteristics of residents in different types of institutions are presented in Chapter 4. The main results on psychiatric morbidity among adults living in institutions are given in Chapter 5.

## 1.5 Plans for later reports

Because of the ambitious nature of the programme of research and the sequential timetables for the four surveys, it is intended to produce a series of reports on different topics or populations, of which this is the fourth (the first dealing with the institutional population). This means that early reports can be produced before all the survey analysis is complete and those interested in specific topics can refer to the relevant report.

The full set of results from the OPCS survey of psychiatric morbidity will be presented in a series of eight reports and four bulletins published from Summer 1995 to Spring 1996. The content of these reports and bulletins are summarised below in the order of the planned publication schedule.

### Private household survey

**Bulletin No.1** *(Published December 1994)*
Prevalence of psychiatric morbidity.

**Report 1** *(Published April 1995)*
Prevalence of psychiatric morbidity by socio-demographic correlates; co-morbidity among psychiatric disorders.

**Report 2** *(Published December 1995)*
Characteristics of people with mental disorders, physical complaints, medication and other forms of treatment, and service use.

**Report 3** *(Published December 1995)*
Difficulties associated with mental disorders in respect of activities of daily living, employment, social functioning, finances. Recent stressful life events and lifestyle behaviours (use of tobacco, alcohol and drugs and their consequences).

### Institutions survey

**Bulletin No. 2** *(Published October 1995)*
Prevalence of psychiatric morbidity in institutions.

**Report 4**
Prevalence of psychiatric morbidity by type of institution.

**Report 5**
Characteristics of people with mental disorders living in institutions, physical complaints, medication, other forms of treatment, and service use within and outside the institution.

**Report 6**
Difficulties associated with mental disorders in respect of activities of daily living, employment, social functioning, finances, recent stressful life events and lifestyle behaviours (use of tobacco, alcohol and drugs and their consequences).

### Survey of homeless people

**Bulletin No. 3**
Prevalence of psychiatric morbidity among homeless people.

**Report 7**
Prevalence of psychiatric morbidity by type of 'accommodation'; physical complaints, medication, other forms of treatment, and service use; difficulties associated with mental disorders in respect of housing, activities of daily living, employment, social functioning, finances. Recent stressful life events and lifestyle behaviours (use of tobacco, alcohol and drugs and their consequences).

### People suffering from a psychotic illness

**Bulletin No. 4**
Summary of the characteristics of people with psychosis.

**Report 8**
Profiles of people with psychosis in terms of differential use of treatment and services.

## Access to the data

Anonymised data from all four surveys will be lodged with the ESRC Data Archive, University of Essex, within 3 months of the publication of the final main report.[4]

## Notes and references

1. *The Health of the Nation: A Strategy for Health in England*, DH, HMSO, 1992

2. *Public Health Information Strategy: Improving Information on Mental Health*, DH, May 1993, Appendix A1, page 29

3. *The Health of the Nation: Key Area Handbook on Mental Illness*, DH, 1993, Section 1.5, page 12.

4. Independent researchers who wish to carry out their own analyses should apply to the Archive for access. For further information about archived data, please contact:

Ms Kathy Sayer
ESRC Data Archive
University of Essex
Wivenhoe Park
Colchester
Essex CO4 3SQ

Tel: (UK) 01206 872323
FAX: (UK) 01206 872003
Email: archive@:Essex.AC.UK.

# 2 Measurement and classification of psychiatric disorders

## 2.1 Choice of measurement instruments

Two different research strategies were used to obtain prevalence estimates of psychiatric morbidity. One approach was used for the major psychiatric disorders (psychotic psychopathology) which can only be assessed reliably by clinically trained interviewers; the other was used for the minor psychiatric disorders (neurotic psychopathology) which are identifiable by lay interviews using structured questionnaires.

### 2.1.1 Psychotic psychopathology

Making assessments of psychotic rather than neurotic disorders is problematic for lay interviewers. A structured questionnaire is too restrictive and a semi-structured questionnaire requires the use of clinical judgements. Therefore, the approach used to assess psychotic psychopathology was to ask OPCS interviewers to find out from residents or staff information about clinical assessment and treatments.

Thus, the process of identifying residents who were suffering from psychotic disorders involved:

- asking residents directly what was the matter with them;

- asking staff, what was the matter with the subject, (if the subject could or would not answer but gave permission for another person to do so);

- asking residents or carers whether subjects were taking anti-psychotic drugs or having anti-psychotic injections;

- establishing whether residents had contact with any health care professional for a mental, nervous or emotional problem

which had been labelled as a psychotic illness.

As this survey focused on people in institutions catering for those with mental illness, it was highly likely that all residents will have had an assessment by a clinician in the recent past.

This approach was different to that used in the private household survey where lay interviewers used the Psychosis Screening Questionnaire to find out if there was any possibility of the subject suffering from a psychotic illness.[1] Psychiatrists were then asked to carry out a follow-up clinical interview.

### 2.1. 2 Neurotic psychopathology

To obtain the diagnoses of neurotic psychopathology, the revised version of the Clinical Interview Schedule (CIS-R) was chosen.[2] Lewis gives the rationale for its use:

> 'Many of the standardised interviews currently used in psychiatry require the interviewer to use expert psychiatric judgements in deciding upon the presence or absence of psychopathology. However, when case definitions are standardised it is customary for clinical judgements to be replaced with rules. The Clinical Interview Schedule was therefore revised, in order to increase standardisation, and to make it suitable for lay interviewers in assessing minor psychiatric disorder in community, general hospital, occupational and primary care research.'

The practical advantages of the CIS-R are:

- it can be administered by non-clinically trained interviewers;

- training in the use of the schedule is straightforward for experienced OPCS interviewers;

5

- length of interview is relatively short (on average, 30 minutes) compared with other methods of assessment.

The CIS-R is made up of 14 sections, each section covering a particular area of neurotic symptoms.

*The 14 Sections of the CIS-R*

Somatic symptoms
Fatigue
Concentration and forgetfulness
Sleep problems
Irritability
Worry about physical health
Depression
Depressive ideas
Worry
Anxiety
Phobias
Panic
Compulsions
Obsessions

Each section within the interview schedule starts with a variable number of mandatory questions which can be regarded as sift or filter questions. They establish the existence of a particular neurotic symptom in the past month. A positive response to these questions leads the interviewer on to further enquiry giving a more detailed assessment of the symptom **in the past week**: frequency, duration, severity and time since onset. It is the answers to these questions which determine the informant's score on each section. More frequent and more severe symptoms result in higher scores.

The minimum score on each section is 0, where the symptom was either not present in the past week or was present only in mild degree. The maximum score on each section is 4 (except for the section on depressive ideas

which has a maximum score of 5), and:

- Summed scores from all 14 sections range between 0 and 57.

- The overall threshold score for significant psychiatric morbidity is 12.

- Symptoms are regarded as severe if they have a score of 2 or more.

The elements which contribute to a score are shown in Appendix B, Part 1. As an illustration, the elements which contribute to a score on the section on Anxiety are shown below.

**Calculation of symptom score for Anxiety from the CIS-R**

|  | Score |
|---|---|
| Felt **generally** anxious/nervous/tense for **4 days or more** in the past seven days... | 1 |
| In past seven days anxiety/nervousness/tension has been **very unpleasant**... | 1 |
| In the past seven days have felt **any of the following symptoms** when anxious/nervous/ tense (Racing heart, sweating or shaking hands, feeling dizzy, difficulty getting one's breath, dry mouth, butterflies in stomach, nausea or wanting to vomit) | 1 |
| Felt anxious/nervous/tense for **more than three hours** in total on any one of the past seven days... | 1 |

Any combination of the elements produce the section score. Diagnoses were obtained by looking at the answers to various sections, including questions which do not necessarily score points, and applying algorithms based on ICD-10 diagnostic criteria[3].

The algorithms for all disorders are shown in Appendix B, Part 2 and the example shown below is for Generalised Anxiety Disorder (GAD).

### Algorithm for GAD

*Conditions which must apply are:*

- Duration greater than six months
- Free-floating anxiety
- Autonomic overactivity
- Overall score on Anxiety section was 2 or more

## 2.2 Classification of disorders for analysis

### Hierarchy of disorders

In this survey, the CIS-R, which was used for clinical assessments of neurotic disorders, covers ICD-10 codes in Sections F3 and F4 only and permits several possible diagnoses to be made. All other disorders, obtained from reports by subjects or staff, could also co-occur with each other or with the neurotic disorders. In order to obtain a **primary diagnosis** hierarchical rules were imposed on the survey data. Psychiatric disorders were subsumed under ICD-10 chapter headings:

### Diagnostic Categories (based on ICD-10)

| | |
|---|---|
| F00 - F09 | Organic Mental Disorders |
| F10 - F19 | Mental and behavioural disorders due to psychoactive substance use |
| F20 - F29 | Schizophrenia, delusional and schizoaffective disorders |
| F30 - F39 | Mood (affective) disorders |
| F40 - F48 | Neurotic, stress-related and somatoform disorders |
| F50 - F59 | Behavioural syndromes associated with physiological disturbances and physical factors |
| F60 - F69 | Disorders of adult personality and behaviour |
| F70 - F79 | Mental retardation |
| F80 - F89 | Disorders of psychological development |
| F90 - F98 | Behavioural and emotional disorders with onset usually occurring in childhood and adolescence |
| Other | Unclassifiable/Insufficient information/No answer |

The rules to obtain the primary diagnosis were in priority order:

1. F00 - F09   Organic mental disorders took precedence over everything else.

2. F20 - F29   Schizophrenia, delusional and schizoaffective disorders took precedence over the remaining groups of disorders.

3. F30 - F39   Affective psychoses, in particular mania and manic depression took precedence over the remaining disorders. Depressive episodes were grouped with neurotic disorders.

4. F40 - F48   Neurotic, stress-related and somatoform disorders took precedence over all others.

When two types of neurotic disorder were found within the category of neurotic disorders, the same rules as those applied in the private household survey were used to obtain the dominant neurotic disorder:

The hierarchical rules were abandoned when the co-occurrence of disorders was examined (See Section 5.2).

| Disorder 1 | Disorder 2 | Priority |
|---|---|---|
| Depressive episode (any severity) | Phobia | Depressive episode (any severity) |
| Depressive episode (mild) | OCD | OCD |
| Depressive episode (moderate) | OCD | Depressive episode (moderate) |
| Depressive episode (severe) | OCD | Depressive episode (severe) |
| Depressive episode (mild) | Panic disorder | Panic disorder |
| Depressive episode (moderate) | Panic disorder | Depressive episode (moderate) |
| Depressive episode (severe) | Panic disorder | Depressive episode (severe) |
| Depressive episode (any severity) | GAD | Depressive episode (any severity) |
| Phobia (any) | OCD | OCD |
| Agoraphobia | GAD | Agoraphobia |
| Social phobia | GAD | Social Phobia |
| Specific phobia | GAD | GAD |
| Panic disorder | OCD | Panic disorder |
| OCD | GAD | OCD |
| Panic disorder | GAD | Panic disorder |

GAD=Generalised Anxiety Disorder
OCD=Obsessive Compulsive Disorder

## Notes and References

1. Bebbington, P.E., and Nayani, T (1995) 'The Psychosis Screening Questionnaire' *International Journal of Methods in Psychiatric Research*, **5**:11-19

2. Lewis, G. and Pelosi, A. J., *Manual of the Revised Clinical Interview Schedule, (CIS-R)* (June 1990) MRC Institute of Psychiatry. Also see Lewis, G, Pelosi, A.J. and Dunn, G., (1992) Measuring Psychiatric disorder in the community: a standardized assessment for use by lay interviewers, *Psychological Medicine*, 22, 465-486

3. *WHO, The ICD-10 Classification of Mental and Behavioural Disorders: Diagnostic Criteria for Research*: 1993, WHO, Geneva.

# 3 Sampling design and interviewing procedures

## 3.1 Introduction

The design of this institutional survey differed from the corresponding private household survey in several key respects. First, to obtain a sample of residents living in institutions which cater for people with mental illness, a sampling frame had to be created that included all such establishments. Second, it was assumed that all residents in these institutions had a mental health problem; hence the CIS-R was used primarily as an instrument for assessment of neurotic disorders rather than screening. Third, the administration of an interview within an institution required different procedures from those used in the private household survey. Procedures had to be developed to obtain information about individuals, many of whom were likely to have difficulty taking part in a lengthy interview.

This chapter describes the creation of the sampling frame and the selection of institutions for the survey, the selection of residents within establishments and the various procedures which were adopted to obtain completed interviews.

## 3.2 Obtaining a sample of institutions

In order to obtain a list of institutions which catered for adults of interest in the survey, a major data gathering exercise was carried out. This involved obtaining the names and addresses of all institutions that provided some sort of medical and/or residential care for adults with mental illness.

The Department of Health, the Scottish Home and Health Department and the Welsh Office were asked to provide lists of places providing particular types of accommodation for adults

with mental health problems. Information was also obtained from the *Hospitals and Health Services Yearbook* and the *Social Services Yearbook.* [1,2]

The information available from these various sources varied in completeness, particularly in respect of the small, unstaffed, group homes or supported accommodation. Therefore, we contacted administrative headquarters of providers of services or support at a local level in an attempt to get complete coverage. Letters were sent to:

a) Directors of Social Services
b) Mental Health Services managers at NHS hospitals
c) Client Service managers at NHS Trusts
d) Directors of appropriate voluntary and charitable organisations
e) Social Work Departments (Scotland)

### Results from the data gathering exercise

A total of 4,295 institutions relevant to the survey were identified from the data-gathering exercise. These were subsumed under 7 broad categories. The categorisation and the number of institutions by type are shown in Table 3.1.

A proportion of institutions in group D, alternative types of residential accommodation, would have been eligible for the Private Household Survey, being unstaffed and having fewer than four permanent residents. Nevertheless, these were also included in this survey.

## 3.3 Sampling institutions

The aim of the sampling design was to interview 1 in 15 of all residents in each type of accommodation. This proportion was felt to

**Table 3.1  Number of institutions catering for people with mental illness by type**

| Category of institution | Number |
|---|---|
| **A  NHS Hospital or Trust** | 430 |
| A1 Large (100+ beds) | 121 |
| A2 Medium (50-99 beds) | 89 |
| A3 Small (<50 beds) | 220 |
| **B  Private Hospital, clinic or nursing home\*** | 105 |
| **C  Residential care homes** | 1,195 |
| C1 Large (10+ beds) | 410 |
| C2 Small (<10 beds) | 785 |
| **D  Alternative types of residential accommodation\*\*** | 2,565 |
| (supervised lodging, group homes and hostels) | |
| **Total number of institutions** | **4,295** |

\*  Private hospitals and clinics in Scotland were included in category A

\*\* Some of these "institutions" would have been eligible for inclusion in the private household survey

give an adequate representation of residents with different disorders. The overall sampling fraction (which takes account of the sampling fraction of institutions and residents) in large residential homes (C1) was originally 1 in 15 but practical issues dictated that the number of interviews in these places was halved.

It was desirable that whenever possible a maximum of 20 interviews should be carried out in medium or large hospitals (50+ residents) and that no more than half the residents should be interviewed in accommodation with 10 or more occupants. A summary of how institutions were sampled is shown in Table 3.2. Sampling residents within selected establishments is described in Section 3.4.

### How cooperation was obtained from the institutions

A different approach was used to gain co-operation from the institution depending on its management structure.

**Table 3.2  Selection and response of institutions**

| | Type of institution\* | | | | | | |
|---|---|---|---|---|---|---|---|
| | A1 | A2 | A3 | B | C1 | C2 | D |
| **No of institutions in each type** | **121** | **89** | **220** | **105** | **410** | **785** | **2,565** |
| Sampling fraction of institutions | 1/2 | 1/3 | 1/6 | 1/5 | 1/15 | 1/15 | 1/15 |
| **No. of selected institutions** | **61** | **29** | **37** | **21** | **28** | **52** | **171** |
| No. of ineligible institutions\*\* | 9 | 10 | 17 | 6 | 2 | 6 | 9 |
| No of refusals of institutions | 4 | 5 | 6 | 6 | 6 | 17 | 88 |
| **No of institutions which cooperated\*\*** | **48** | **14** | **14** | **9** | **20** | **29** | **74** |

\*  The description of each type is shown in Table 3.1

\*\* The total number of institutions selected for the survey was 399 and 208 cooperated.

For NHS accommodation, private hospitals, nursing homes and clinics, letters asking for co-operation were sent to the general manager or the mental heath services manager at that institution.

To gain access to residential care homes, the Director of Social Services was contacted, as well as the home itself. For other types of residential homes (mostly unstaffed), the governing authorities who had responsibility for the residents were written to.

### Acceptance and contact sheet

Each of the 399 sampled institutions was sent an **Acceptance and Contact sheet** which asked for the following information:

- the number of permanently resident adults aged 16-64;

- the name, position and telephone number of the contact person at the establishment;

- the name and address of other interested parties.

A permanent resident was defined as:

(a)  living in the sampled establishment for the past 6 months;

(b)  living in the sampled establishment for less than 6 months but:

(i)  had been living in residential accommodation for the past 6 months, or

(ii)  had no other permanent address, or

(iii)  was likely to stay in the establishment for the foreseeable future.

Institutions which did not respond to our enquiries or did not return an acceptance sheet were followed up by an interviewer. However, this procedure was not enforced for unstaffed

accommodation so as not to cause distress to residents who did not want to participate.

### Ineligible institutions

Table 3.2 shows that 59 of the 399 selected institutions were ineligible for the survey and consequently withdrawn. The main reason for ineligibility was that the institutions were acute units and did not fulfil the survey's criteria of having 'permanent residents'. Other reasons for exclusion were that the institution catered for people aged 65 or over or for those who were mentally handicapped rather than mentally ill.

### Non-response by institutions

There were very few refusals among the hospitals, clinics, nursing homes and residential care homes. The main reasons for these refusals were that some institutions were in the midst of major administrative changes or those in charge were worried by safety considerations.

The largest proportions of losses came from the alternative types of residential care: supported lodging, unstaffed group homes and hostels. Here the losses were mainly non-contacts rather than refusals. It was difficult to negotiate access to accommodation where staff were not living on the premises.

## 3.4 Sampling residents

The aim of the sampling design was to interview 1 in 15 of all residents in each type of accommodation, except for large residential homes where the target was to interview 1 in 30 residents. *(Table 3.3)*

Table 3.3 shows that once access to establishment had been agreed, about 11% of residents refused to take part. In hospitals, nursing homes and residential care homes, the main reason for refusing was that the residents themselves were incapable of carrying out the interview and a

11

**Table 3.3  Sampling of residents**

| Type of institution* | A1 | A2 | A3 | B | C1 | C2 | D |
|---|---|---|---|---|---|---|---|
| Overall sampling fraction | 1/15 | 1/15 | 1/15 | 1/15 | 1/30 | 1/15 | 1/15 |
| Sampling fraction of institutions | 1/2 | 1/3 | 1/6 | 1/5 | 1/15 | 1/15 | 1/15 |
| Sampling fraction of residents | 2/15 | 1/5 | 2/5 | 1/3 | 1/2 | 1/1 | 1/1 |
| **No. of selected residents\*\*** | **470** | **121** | **83** | **60** | **151** | **167** | **276** |
| No. of refusals of residents | 54 | 14 | 10 | 2 | 17 | 11 | 40 |
| **No. of residents who co-operated\*\*** | **416** | **107** | **73** | **58** | **134** | **156** | **236** |

\*  The description of each type of institution is shown in Table 3.1
\*\* The total number of residents selected for the survey was 1,328 and 1,180 cooperated.

proxy informant could not be found. In smaller establishments, residents were worried about being classified as having psychiatric problems. Many were on their way to reintegrating themselves into the community and did not want to be labelled as having a mental health problem.

The survey data were weighted for differential non-response in each type of establishment and for the disproportionately lower chances of selection in large residential care homes. Full details are given in Appendix A.

## 3.5 Organisation of the interview

The interviewing procedures are shown in the flow chart (*Figure 3.1*).

Thus, every sampled adult was asked Schedule A which covered:

- Socio-demographic characteristics
- General health questions
- Clinical Interview Schedule - Revised (CIS-R)
- The Psychosis Screening Questionnaire (PSQ) and associated questions which indicate the possibility of psychotic disorders

Unlike the private household survey, where an above-threshold score or a positive screen on the PSQ dictated what happened next, all individuals in the institutional survey were asked Schedule B which was made up of 10 sections:

- Long standing illness
- Medication and treatment
- Health, Social and Voluntary care services
- Activities of daily living and informal care
- Recent stressful life events
- Social activities, social networks and social support
- Education and employment
- Finances
- Smoking
- Alcohol consumption

All subjects were also given a self completion questionnaire (D) covering alcohol dependency. This was an abridged version of the one used in the private household survey. Questions were omitted on problems resulting from alcohol consumption, and dependency and problems as a result of the use of drugs. The questions dealing with these topics were deemed inappropriate for residents of institutions.

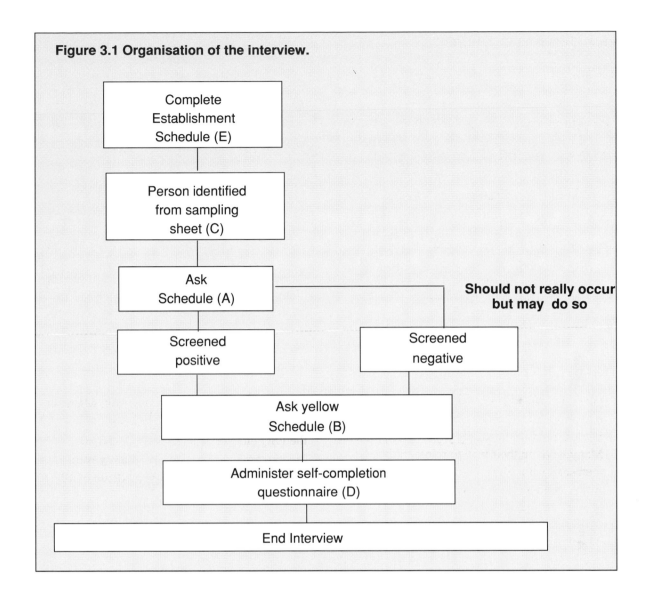

**Figure 3.1 Organisation of the interview.**

Complete Establishment Schedule (E)

Person identified from sampling sheet (C)

Ask Schedule (A)

**Should not really occur but may do so**

Screened positive

Screened negative

Ask yellow Schedule (B)

Administer self-completion questionnaire (D)

End Interview

## 3.6 Interviewing procedures

### Introducing the survey

In introducing the survey interviewers were told to avoid terms such as 'psychiatric morbidity' and 'the mentally ill', whether talking to the contact person or the informant. Even though the sample for this survey was selected because they were known to be living in accommodation for people with mental health problems, it was still felt that words had to be chosen very carefully. Interviewers were instructed:

'Some people with mental illness may be willing to confide in medical professionals about a mental health problem but they be more reticent with other people. There are various reasons for this denial: stigma, embarrassment, perceived consequences for employment or housing opportunities. Some of the sample may be people who feel they have got over their mental health problem and are in the process of reintegrating themselves back into the community. Tread cautiously. Concentrate on using the expression, strains and stresses of everyday life. This is something most people even in hospitals, nursing homes or residential accommodation can relate to.'[1]

## Mental state of informant

It was anticipated that some of the sampled residents would have a severe psychiatric problem. However, as residents of institutions, they were likely to be known to at least one of the health, social and voluntary care services; even those in unstaffed lodging or group homes. Because of this contact, most sampled residents were having treatment and interviewers were told to wait for periods of lucidity in subjects before carrying out an interview.

## Finding out if the informant could be interviewed

The contact person at the institution was asked whether the sampled resident was capable of being interviewed. A blank schedule was shown to the contact person for this purpose. At the same time s/he was asked about who could give the most reliable information about medication, treatment or use of services.

## Proxy interviews

If the informant could not be interviewed during the field period the proxy interview procedure was carried out. Wherever possible, interviewers tried to get the informant's permission to carry this out. If the interview was felt to be a strain on the informant, it was split: Schedule A with the informant and Schedule B with a proxy, if a proxy informant was available.

In some of the unstaffed and supported accommodation, there were occasions when there was not anyone who could be called upon to act as a proxy informant. In some hospitals, homes and clinics staff were extremely busy. Questions were never asked of co-residents.

## Privacy

Wherever possible, interviews were carried out in privacy. Sometimes, the availability of space in the institution for an interview was limited. On other occasions, staff insisted that safety considerations took precedence over the desire for privacy.

## Notes and references

1. *The Hospitals and Health Services Yearbook,* 1993. The Institute of Health Services Management, William Clowes Ltd, Beccles and London.

2. *Social Services Yearbook,* 1993, Pitman Publishing, London.

3. OPCS, *Survey of Health and Well-being, Instructions for Interviewers,* 1993.

# 4 Distribution of residents among institutions

## 4.1 Hospitals and residential accommodation

Although the sampling design involved a seven-fold classification of institutions, this categorisation was verified with the contact person at each institution and a more detailed breakdown was produced. About a third of the sampled residents were long-stay NHS hospital patients, a quarter were in residential care homes, another third in alternative forms of residential care, and the smallest group (7%) were residing in private hospitals, clinics or nursing homes. Table 4.1 also shows how these proportions translate into grossed estimates, that is, estimates of the total number permanent resident in each type of institution based on sampling fractions and response to the interview. (*Table 4.1*)

## Table 4.1 Numbers and proportions of residents by type of institution

| | Grossed estimates | Number of residents | Proportion of residents |
|---|---|---|---|
| | | | % |
| **NHS Hospital or Trust** | **11,300** | **407** | **34** |
| Psychiatric hospital | 9,500 | 341 | 29 |
| Psychiatric unit/ward of general hospital | 1,800 | 66 | 6 |
| **Private hospital, clinic or nursing home** | **2,200** | **80** | **7** |
| **Residential care home** | **8,300** | **297** | **25** |
| **Alternative types of residential accommodation** | **11,400** | **408** | **34** |
| Group Home | 4,600 | 165 | 14 |
| Hostel | 4,200 | 125 | 10 |
| Recognised lodging or ordinary housing | 2,600 | 95 | 8 |
| Sheltered community | 500 | 19 | 2 |
| **Unclassifiable** | **100** | **4** | **0** |
| **All institutions** | **33,200** | **1,191** | **100** |

## 4.2 Residential care homes

About a third of sampled residents in residential care homes were in accommodation which provided medical or nursing care, rehabilitative support services and counselling for independent living or jobs. This includes services available in the institution and those brought in from outside. About a third of residents were living in institutions which provided two of these three range of services, the majority provided with rehabilitation services and counselling. The remaining residents received just one of these services. (*Table 4.2*)

## Table 4.2 Services provided to residents in sampled institutions

| Type of service mix | Proportion of residents |
|---|---|
| | % |
| Medical and nursing care & Rehabilitative support services & Counselling for jobs/ independent living | 34 |
| Medical and nursing care & Rehabilitative support services services | 6 |
| Medical and nursing care & Counselling for jobs/independent living | 4 |
| Rehabilitative support services & Counselling for jobs/independent living | 22 |
| Medical and nursing care only | 10 |
| Rehabilitative support services only | 15 |
| Counselling for jobs/independent living only | 9 |
| *Base (All residents)* | *1,191* |

Residents in local authority care homes were more likely than others to have medical or nursing care available to them. People living in residential care homes run by voluntary or charitable organisations were more likely than those in LA- or privately-run establishments to have access to counselling for independent living or jobs. (*Figure 4.1*)

## 4.3 Alternative types of residential accommodation

The tenfold classification of alternative types of alternative residential accommodation was taken from Wing's paper on assessment of needs.[1] The description and definition of each type is given below:

*Ordinary housing or recognised lodging*

*Unsupervised in ordinary housing* with a degree of protection, eg from eviction if in rent arrears.

*Supervised in ordinary housing* with regular domiciliary supervision of personal care, household maintenance, hygiene safety and rent payments.

*Recognised lodging* where the landlady has been selected for qualities of kindness and standard of care, Supervises personal care, hygiene, safety and rent payments.

*Group homes*

*Unsupervised group home* where a group of people live together in an ordinary house, with protected rent and occasional visits.

*Supervised group home* where a group of people live together in an ordinary house but have regular (up to daily) visits by housekeeper for household maintenance. No care staff live in.

*Clustered group homes* where a warden lives nearby and makes regular domiciliary checks.

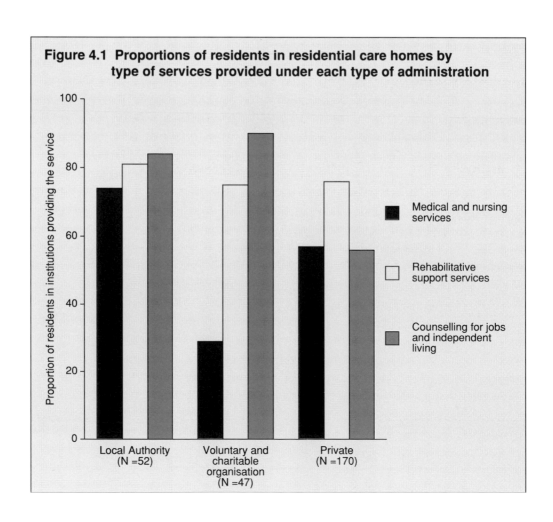

**Figure 4.1 Proportions of residents in residential care homes by type of services provided under each type of administration**

Proportion of residents in institutions providing the service

- Medical and nursing services
- Rehabilitative support services
- Counselling for jobs and independent living

Local Authority (N =52)

Voluntary and charitable organisation (N =47)

Private (N =170)

**Table 4.3  Proportions of residents in different types of alternative residential accommodation**

|  | Number of residents | Proportion of residents |
|---|---|---|
|  |  | % |
| **Ordinary housing or recognised lodging** | **95** | **23** |
|  |  |  |
| Unsupervised | 26 | 6 |
| Supervised | 53 | 13 |
| Recognised lodging | 16 | 4 |
|  |  |  |
| **Group homes** | **165** | **41** |
|  |  |  |
| Unsupervised | 60 | 15 |
| Supervised | 83 | 20 |
| Clustered group homes | 22 | 6 |
|  |  |  |
| **Hostels** | **125** | **31** |
|  |  |  |
| Supervised | 117 | 29 |
| Higher supervision | 8 | 2 |
| Intensive supervision | 0 | - |
|  |  |  |
| **Sheltered community** | **19** | **5** |
|  |  |  |
| **Other** | **4** | **1** |
|  |  |  |
| *All* | *408* | *100* |

Some are built around a quadrangle with entrance by warden's flat.

### Hostels

*Supervised hostel* where care staff live in and are on call at night. Provide regular domiciliary supervision.

*Higher supervision hostel* where care staff are in attendance all night.

*Intensive supervision hostel* with higher staff levels than above. For people with severe behaviour disturbance or disability.

### Sheltered community

The largest group of sampled residents in alternative forms of residential accommodation were in group homes (40%) and about a half of the residents had daily supervision. *(Table 4.3)*

**Table 4.4  Institutional or private household status of residents in all**

|  | Ordinary housing or recognised lodging | Group homes | Hostels | Sheltered community | Other |
|---|---|---|---|---|---|
|  | % | % | % | % | % |
| Private household population | 81 | 79 | 4 | [-] | [-] |
|  |  |  |  |  |  |
| Institutional population | 7 | 7 | 96 | [19] | [-] |
|  |  |  |  |  |  |
| Not known | 12 | 15 | - | [-] | [4] |
| *Base* | *95* | *165* | *125* | *19* | *4* |

### 4.4 Overlap between the institutional and private household surveys

Some forms of residential accommodation (see Section 4.2), especially the ordinary housing, recognised lodging, and group homes, could also be classified as private households according to the standard definition used in OPCS household surveys.[2]

The definition of a household is:

> 'one person or a group of people who have the accommodation as their **only** or **main** residence **AND** (for a group of people) **either** share at least one meal a day **or** share the living accommodation'

Table 4.4 shows that approximately 80% of all residents living in recognised housing or group homes were part of the private household population. However, practically all hostel residents were part of the institutional population. Although not shown in the table, the degree of supervision in the recognised lodging and group homes seemed to make little difference to the split between those classified as institutions or private households.

All the people living in residential accommodation sampled in the institutional survey are included in the analysis shown in this report.

### Notes and References

1 Wing, J.K. and Furlong, R. (1986) A haven for the severely disabled within the context of a comprehensive psychiatric service, *British Journal of psychiatry,* **149**, 449-57

2 McCrossan, L., (1991) *A handbook for interviewers: A manual of Social Survey practice and procedures on structured interviewing*, HMSO, London

# 5 Prevalence of psychiatric disorders

## 5.1 Introduction

This chapter presents the main survey estimates of the numbers and prevalence rates of psychiatric disorders among residents of establishments catering primarily for those suffering from mental health problems.

The categorisation of psychiatric disorder shown in the tables in this chapter is very different from that used in the private household survey because of the higher prevalence of the more severe psychopathologies in institutions[1].

The characteristics of the establishments used in the analysis in this chapter are shown in Figure 5.1.

## 5.2 Estimates of psychopathology by type of institution.

More than two thirds of the adults aged 16 to 64 interviewed in establishments catering for people with mental health problems were found to be suffering from schizophrenia, delusional or schizo-affective disorders, representing 23,100 individuals out of a total estimated establishment population of 33,200. The next most common disorder category, the neurotic, stress-related and somatoform disorders, affected 8% of residents, representing fewer than three thousand individuals.

Eight percent of individuals suffered from an affective psychoses, again representing fewer than three thousand individuals in the institutional population. It should be noted that diagnoses of depressive episode are included in the category of neurotic disorders and not affective psychoses. Also, no individuals were classified as suffering from mental retardation.

The survey specifically excluded institutions catering primarily for those with this disorder. *(Table 5.1)*

As indicated in Chapter 4, institutions catering primarily for those with mental health problems can be grouped for analytic purposes into two broad categories: hospitals and residential accommodation. The latter category includes residential care homes as well as alternative types of residential care. There were several obvious differences between the two settings in the distribution of psychiatric disorders. The prevalence of schizophrenia and related disorders was significantly higher (p<0.01) in hospitals than in residential accommodation: about three quarters of those in hospitals were found to be suffering from this group of disorders compared with two thirds of those in residential care. The prevalence of mood disorders at 10% was also significantly higher in hospitals (p<0.01). Conversely, the prevalence of neurotic, stress-related and somatoform disorders was found to be three times higher among those in residential care than among those in hospitals (p<0.01) .*(Table 5.2)*

The hospitals, clinics and nursing homes were grouped into three categories: NHS psychiatric hospital, NHS unit or ward of general hospital, and private hospital, clinic or nursing home. Again the distribution of the two largest categories of disorder varied by type of institution, with the clearest difference being observed between the private establishments and the NHS hospitals. The prevalence of schizophrenia and related disorders was significantly higher in the NHS psychiatric hospitals and in the NHS units or wards than in the private institutions (p<0.01). The prevalence of the affective psychoses was conversely significantly higher in the private establishments than in the NHS establishments: about one in four of those in private hospitals, clinics or homes were found

**Figure 5.1  Characteristics of institutions used in analysis**

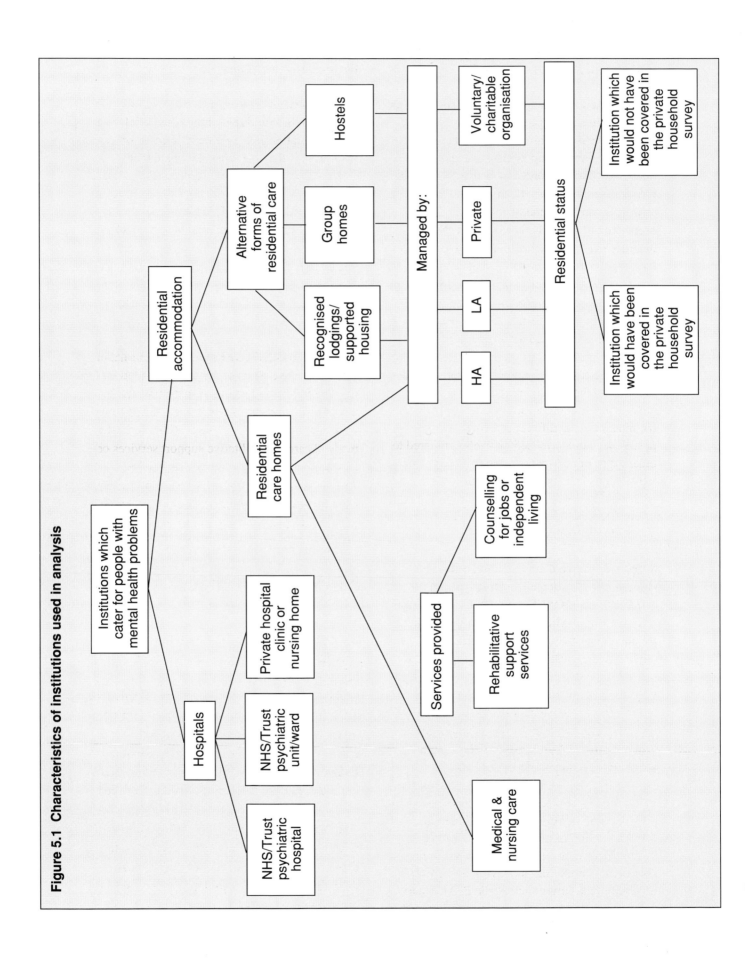

to be suffering from affective psychoses compared to about one in twelve of those in NHS hospitals (p<0.01) *(Table 5.3).*

The prevalence of the psychiatric disorders was also examined by type of residential care setting. About two thirds of residents of residential care and group homes, and about three quarters of those in ordinary housing or recognised lodgings, were suffering from schizophrenia and related disorders. The proportion of individuals with this type of disorder in hostels was significantly lower than the proportion in other residential accommodation (p<0.01). Similarly, the proportion in ordinary housing/recognised housing was significantly higher than in other types of residential accommodation (p<0.01).

There were small differences between the types of residential care accommodation in the prevalence of neurosis and related disorders, the most obvious difference being the higher prevalence among those in hostels compared to other types of accommodation (p<0.01). The prevalence of this group of disorders was also significantly lower in ordinary housing/recognised lodgings than in other types of establishment (p<0.0). *(Table 5.4).*

When interviewing at residential care homes and places providing alternative types of residential care, OPCS interviewers also sought information on who managed or supported the establishment: whether it was a Health Authority or Trust, Local Authority, voluntary or charitable organisation, was privately run or was run by some other organisation. The prevalence of the psychiatric disorders was found to differ with the management of the organisation. The proportion of those with schizophrenia and related disorders was significantly higher in the accommodation run by Health Authorities or Local Authorities than in the private or voluntary/charitable sector homes. Around three quarters of residents in the HA/LA run accommodation were in this disorder category compared with under two thirds in the accommodation run by voluntary/ charitable organisations (p<0.01). In contrast the proportion of those with neuroses and

related disorders is slightly higher in the homes managed or supported by voluntary or charitable organisations. *(Table 5.5)*

OPCS interviewers were asked to record whether they would regard the residential accommodation as a private household or as an institution if they had been allocated that address from the Postcode Address File while interviewing on the private household survey of psychiatric morbidity. This gives an indication of whether the accommodation more closely approximates to an institution or a private household. The distribution of psychiatric disorders by type of accommodation however showed that the prevalence of each disorder was similar for both types. *(Table 5.6)*

Only in residential care homes was information sought as to the types of services provided for residents. The proportion of those with each disorder did not vary significantly with the type of services offered by the institution: formal medical care, rehabilitative support services or counselling for jobs or independent living. Around two thirds of residents were suffering from schizophrenia while around one in eight had a neurotic disorder. *(Table 5.7)*

## 5.3 Comorbidity of psychiatric disorders

Comorbidity between the psychiatric disorders was examined for people suffering from schizophrenia; this group was chosen for analysis as it comprised almost three-quarters of all disorders in institutions. The most common other disorders of these individuals were examined according to whether the individual had no other disorder, one other disorder, two other disorders or three or more other disorders.

Over half of individuals with schizophrenia and related disorders had no other disorder while over a quarter had one other disorder, most commonly generalised anxiety disorder (6%) or manic depression (5%). About one in ten of those with schizophrenia and related disorders

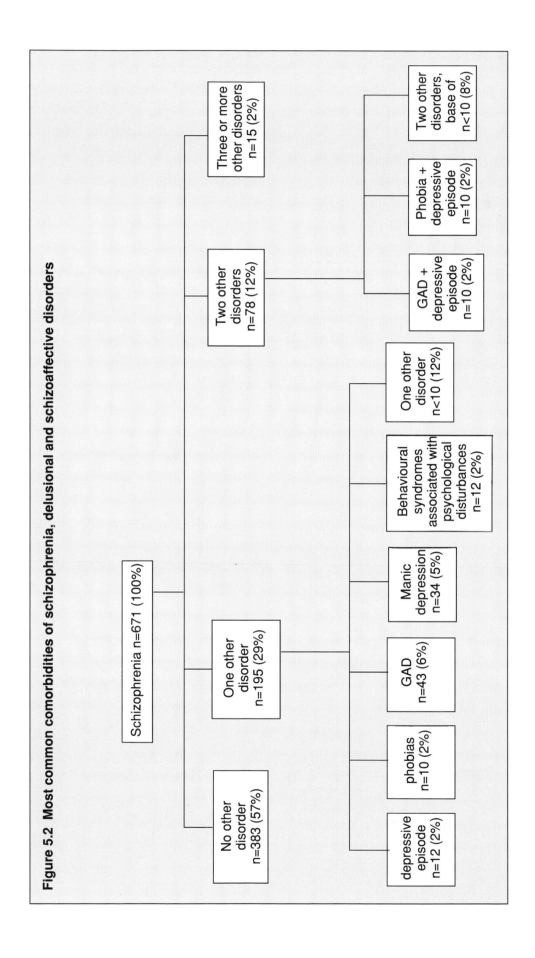

Figure 5.2 Most common comorbidities of schizophrenia, delusional and schizoaffective disorders

also had two other disorders, with generalised anxiety disorder plus depressive episode or phobia plus depressive episode occurring most frequently (though actual percentages in these groups are low). Those suffering from three or more disorders made up only a small percentage of the total (2%). *(Figure 5.2)*

It should be noted that psychotic diagnoses were likely to be given as a primary diagnosis, with no secondary diagnosis even when one exists. Although, attempts were made to get CIS-R data for all selected residents, about a quarter of the sample could not be interviewed. In these cases proxy information was obtained.

## Notes and references

1. Meltzer, H., Gill, B., Petticrew, and Hinds, K., (1995) *The OPCS Surveys of Psychiatric Morbidity in Great Britain, Report 1, The prevalence of psychiatric morbidity among adults aged 16-64 living in private households in Great Britain*, HMSO London

**Table 5.1  Grossed estimates and proportions of residents with each type of disorder**

|  |  | Grossed estimates * | SE | % |
|---|---|---|---|---|
| **Primary diagnosis (based on ICD-10)** | | | | |
| F00-F09 | Organic mental disorders | 600 | 200 | 2 |
| F10-F19 | Mental and behavioural disorders due to psychoactive substance use | 200 | 100 | 1 |
| F20-F29 | Schizophrenia, delusional and schizoaffective disorders | 23,100 | 700 | 70 |
| F30-F39 | Mood disorders excluding depressive episode: affective psychoses | 2,700 | 500 | 8 |
| F40-F48 | Neurotic, stress-related and somatoform disorders including depressive episode | 2,800 | 500 | 8 |
| F50-F59 | Behavioural syndromes associated with psychological disturbances and physical factors | 300 | 100 | 1 |
| F60-F69 | Disorders of adult personality and behaviour | 200 | 100 | 0 |
| F70-F79 | Mental retardation | - | - | - |
| F80-F89 | Disorders of psychological development | 400 | 200 | 1 |
| F90-F98 | Behavioural and emotional disorders with onset usually occurring in childhood and adolescence | 0 | 0 | 0 |
|  | Insufficient information | 2,600 | - | 8 |
|  | No answer / refusal | 400 | - | 1 |
| *Base (all residents)* | | *33,200* | | *100* |

* rounded to nearest 100

24

**Table 5.2 Proportions of residents in hospitals and residential accommodation with each type of disorder**

|  |  | Hospitals | Residential accommodation | All accommodation |
|---|---|---|---|---|
| **Primary diagnosis (based on ICD-10)** |  | % | % | % |
| F00-F09 | Organic mental disorders | 3 | 0 | 2 |
| F10-F19 | Mental and behavioural disorders due to psychoactive substance use | 0 | 1 | 0 |
| F20-F29 | Schizophrenia, delusional and schizoaffective disorders | 74 | 67 | 70 |
| F30-F39 | Mood disorders excluding depressive episode: affective psychoses | 10 | 6 | 8 |
| F40-F48 | Neurotic, stress-related and somatoform disorders including depressive episode | 4 | 12 | 8 |
| F50-F59 | Behavioural syndromes associated with psychological disturbances and physical factors | 1 | 0 | 1 |
| F60-F69 | Disorders of adult personality and behaviour | 0 | 0 | 0 |
| F70-F79 | Mental retardation | 0 | 0 | 0 |
| F80-F89 | Disorders of psychological development | 0 |  |  |
| F90-F98 | Behavioural and emotional disorders with onset usually occurring in childhood and adolescence | 0 | 0 | 1 |
|  | Insufficient information | 5 | 10 | 8 |
|  | No answer / refusal | 1 | 2 | 1 |
| *Base (all residents)* |  | *486* | *705* | *1,191* |

**Table 5.3  Proportions of residents with each type of disorder by type of hospital setting**

| | | NHS psychiatric hospital | NHS unit/ward of general hospital | Private hospital, clinic or nursing home | All hospitals, clinics, or nursing homes |
|---|---|---|---|---|---|
| **Primary diagnosis (based on ICD-10)** | | % | % | % | % |
| F00-F09 | Organic mental disorders | 4 | 1 | 1 | 2 |
| F10-F19 | Mental and behavioural disorders due to psychoactive substance use | 0 | 0 | 0 | 0 |
| F20-F29 | Schizophrenia, delusional and schizoaffective disorders | 75 | 81 | 61 | 72 |
| F30-F39 | Mood disorders excluding depressive episode: affective psychoses | 7 | 10 | 24 | 14 |
| F40-F48 | Neurotic, stress-related and somatoform disorders including depressive episode | 4 | 3 | 4 | 4 |
| F50-F59 | Behavioural syndromes associated with psychological disturbances and physical factors | 0 | 2 | 5 | 2 |
| F60-F69 | Disorders of adult personality and behaviour | 1 | 0 | 0 | 0 |
| F70-F79 | Mental retardation | 0 | 0 | 0 | 0 |
| F80-F89 | Disorders of psychological development | 0 | 0 | 3 | 1 |
| F90-F98 | Behavioural and emotional disorders with onset usually occurring in childhood and adolescence | 0 | 0 | 0 | 0 |
| | Insufficient information | 6 | 3 | 0 | 3 |
| | No answer / refusal | 1 | 0 | 1 | 0 |
| *Base (all residents)* | | *341* | *66* | *80* | *487* |

**Table 5.4  Proportions of residents with each type of disorder by type of residential accommodation**

| | | Residential care home | Group home | Hostels | Ordinary/ recognised housing | All residential accommodation |
|---|---|---|---|---|---|---|
| **Primary diagnosis (based on ICD-10)** | | % | % | % | % | % |
| F00-F09 | Organic mental disorders | 1 | 0 | 0 | 0 | 0 |
| F10-F19 | Mental and behavioural disorders due to psychoactive substance use | 1 | 1 | 0 | 2 | 1 |
| F20-F29 | Schizophrenia, delusional and schizoaffective disorders | 65 | 68 | 58 | 76 | 67 |
| F30-F39 | Mood disorders excluding depressive episode: affective psychoses | 7 | 9 | 3 | 6 | 6 |
| F40-F48 | Neurotic, stress-related and somatoform disorders including depressive episode | 11 | 11 | 19 | 7 | 12 |
| F50-F59 | Behavioural syndromes associated with psychological disturbances and physical factors | 1 | 0 | 0 | 0 | 0 |
| F60-F69 | Disorders of adult personality and behaviour | 1 | 1 | 0 | 0 | 0 |
| F70-F79 | Mental retardation | 0 | 0 | 0 | 0 | 0 |
| F80-F89 | Disorders of psychological development | 2 | 0 | 2 | 2 | 2 |
| F90-F98 | Behavioural and emotional disorders with onset usually occurring in childhood and adolescence | 0 | 0 | 0 | 0 | 0 |
| | Insufficient information | 10 | 8 | 16 | 6 | 10 |
| | No answer / refusal | 1 | 3 | 2 | 1 | 2 |
| *Base (all residents)* | | *297* | *166* | *125* | *94* | *705* |

**Table 5.5  Proportions of residents with each type of disorder in residential care home by who manages the accommodation***

| Primary diagnosis (based on ICD-10) | | Health authority | Local authority | Privately run | Voluntary/ charitable organisation |
|---|---|---|---|---|---|
| | | % | % | % | % |
| F00-F09 | Organic mental disorders | 0 | 0 | 1 | 0 |
| F10-F19 | Mental and behavioural disorders due to psychoactive substance use | 2 | 0 | 1 | 1 |
| F20-F29 | Schizophrenia, delusional and schizoaffective disorders | 74 | 77 | 63 | 60 |
| F30-F39 | Mood disorders excluding depressive episode: affective psychoses | 9 | 5 | 7 | 8 |
| F40-F48 | Neurotic, stress-related and somatoform disorders including depressive episode | 8 | 12 | 12 | 16 |
| F50-F59 | Behavioural syndromes associated with psychological disturbances and physical factors | 0 | 0 | 1 | 0 |
| F60-F69 | Disorders of adult personality and behaviour | 0 | 2 | 0 | 0 |
| F70-F79 | Mental retardation | 0 | 0 | 0 | 0 |
| F80-F89 | Disorders of psychological development | 0 | 0 | 2 | 0 |
| F90-F98 | Behavioural and emotional disorders with onset usually occurring in childhood and adolescence | 0 | 0 | 0 | 0 |
| | Insufficient information | 6 | 4 | 12 | 13 |
| | No answer / refusal | 2 | 1 | 2 | 2 |
| *Base (all residents)* | | *72* | *187* | *480* | *232* |

* Institutions with joint administration are included in both columns.

**Table 5.6 Proportions of residents with each type of disorder in residential accommodation by status of institution**

| | | Residential accommodation as institutions | Residential accommodation as private households | All |
|---|---|---|---|---|
| **Primary diagnosis (based on ICD-10)** | | % | % | % |
| F00-F09 | Organic mental disorders | 1 | 1 | 1 |
| F10-F19 | Mental and behavioural disorders due to psychoactive substance use | 0 | 2 | 1 |
| F20-F29 | Schizophrenia, delusional and schizoaffective disorders | 65 | 68 | 66 |
| F30-F39 | Mood disorders excluding depressive episode: affective psychoses | 6 | 8 | 7 |
| F40-F48 | Neurotic, stress-related and somatoform disorders including depressive episode | 13 | 10 | 11 |
| F50-F59 | Behavioural syndromes associated with psychological disturbances and physical factors | 1 | 0 | 0 |
| F60-F69 | Disorders of adult personality and behaviour | 0 | 0 | 0 |
| F70-F79 | Mental retardation | 0 | 0 | 0 |
| F80-F89 | Disorders of psychological development | 2 | 1 | 2 |
| F90-F98 | Behavioural and emotional disorders with onset usually occurring in childhood and adolescence | 0 | 0 | 0 |
| | Insufficient information | 11 | 9 | 10 |
| | No answer / refusal | 2 | 3 | 2 |
| *Base (all residents)* | | *406* | *239* | *645* |

**Table 5.7  Proportions of residents with each type of disorder by services provided by their institutions***

| | Medical and nursing staff | Rehabilitative support services | Counselling for independent living/jobs |
|---|---|---|---|
| **Primary diagnosis (based on ICD-10)** | % | % | % |
| F00-F09  Organic mental disorders | 1 | 1 | 0 |
| F10-F19  Mental and behavioural disorders due to psychoactive substance use | 0 | 1 | 1 |
| F20-F29  Schizophrenic, delusional and schizoaffective disorders | 61 | 66 | 63 |
| F30-F39  Mood disorders excluding depressive episode: affective psychoses | 6 | 6 | 7 |
| F40-F48  Neurotic, stress-related and somatoform disorders including depressive episode | 14 | 11 | 13 |
| F50-F59  Behavioural syndromes associated with psychological disturbances and physical factors | 0 | 1 | 1 |
| F60-F69  Disorders of adult personality and behaviour | 2 | 1 | 1 |
| F70-F79  Mental retardation | 0 | 0 | 0 |
| F80-F89  Disorders of psychological development | 4 | 2 | 2 |
| F90-F98  Behavioural and emotional disorders with onset usually occurring in childhood and adolescence | 0 | 0 | 0 |
| Insufficient information | 11 | 10 | 11 |
| No answer / refusal | 2 | 1 | 1 |
| *Base (all residents)* | *162* | *228* | *206* |

* Many institutions provide more than one service

# Appendix A  Sampling, non-response and weighting

## A.1  Sampling of individuals within institutions

A sample of adults was selected in a relatively large number of hospitals and in residential homes where the total number of beds was ten or more. This was done in preference to interviewing all eligible residents because:

a)  it helped interviewers get in and out of the institution fairly quickly causing minium disruption to the routine of the staff;

b)  individuals within institutions will tend to be similar to each other whereas those in different institutions differ markedly from one another. Taking many residents of a few institutions can lead to a substantial increase in standard errors around survey estimates. Sampling took place in over 200 institutions.

### *Selection procedure*

The selection procedure carried out in the institution was as follows:

(i)  The interviewers listed all 'permanent residents' who were aged 16–64 according to an easily available criterion (ward, room number, age), ie, in a systematic way.  Each eligible person was assigned a person number.

(ii)  The person to be interviewed was then defined by reference to a selection sheet which had a list of person numbers based on the sampling fraction already defined for that particular institution.

The selection sheet was based on information supplied by the institution of the number of potential, eligible respondents.

The number of persons identified by the institution was not always identical to that found by the interviewer after a rigorous application of the eligibility criteria. Nevertheless, the sampling fraction was adhered to as long as the difference was not vastly different. If there was a considerable difference the sampling fraction was adjusted up or down to obtain the expected number of interviews at the institution.

## A.2  Weighting for non-response and institution size

Weighting occurred in four steps to take account of

1.  ineligible institutions within strata;

2.  the different probabilities of selecting establishments within strata.;

3.  the cooperation of informants within institutions;

4.  the different probabilities of selecting residents within institutions.

These four elements constitute the four expressions in the equation below. Note that a weighting factor was calculated for each institution.

$$W_k = \frac{s\,(e) - i\,(e)}{r\,(e)} * \frac{P\,(e)}{S\,(e)} * \frac{\Sigma S_k\,(p)}{\Sigma r_k\,(p)} * \frac{1}{f_k\,(p)}$$

where...

$W_k$  = weighting factor for each institution
$s(e)$  =  the set sample of institutions
$i(e)$  =  ineligible institutions

r(e)  = co-operating institutions

P(e)  = population of institutions

S(e)  = set sample of institutions

$S_k(p)$ = set sample of residents within institution k

$r_k(p)$  = co-operating residents in institution k

$f_k(p)$  = sampling fraction of residents within institutions

The assumptions made in using the formula are:

- the proportion of eligible institutions of different types in the same as the population is the proportion in the set sample;

- all non-respondents are eligible;
- using the overall response rate for people within institutions at the stratum level rather than the institution level, as some of the institutions have very small sample sizes.

After the weights were applied, the weighted sample size differed from the actual (pre-weighting) sample size. A final weighting factor was therefore applied to correct the change in the base. This returned the weighted sample size to its original size.

# Appendix B  Psychiatric measurement

## B.1 Calculation of CIS-R symptom scores

### Fatigue
Scores relate to fatigue or feeling tired or lacking in energy in the past week.
*Score one for each of:*
- Symptom present on four days or more
- Symptom present for more than three hours in total on any day
- Subject had to push him/herself to get things done on at least one occasion
- Symptom present when subject doing things he/she enjoys or used to enjoy at least once

### Sleep problems
Scores relate to problems with getting to sleep, or otherwise, with sleeping more than is usual for the subject in the past week.
*Score one for each of:*
- Had problems with sleep for four nights or more
- Spent at least 1 hour trying to get to sleep on the night with least sleep
- Spent at least 1 hour trying to get to sleep on the night with least sleep
- Spent 3 hours or more truing to get to sleep on four nights or more
- Slept for at least 1 hour longer than usual for subject on any night
- Slept for at least 1 hour longer than usual for subject on any night
- Slept for more than 3 hours longer than usual for subject on four nights or more

### Irritability
Scores relate to feelings of irritability, being short-tempered or angry in the past week.
*Score one for each of:*
- Symptom present for four days or more
- Symptom present for more than 1 hour on any day
- Wanted to shout at someone in past week (even if subject had not actually shouted)
- Had arguments, rows or quarrels or lost temper with someone and felt it was unjustified on at least one occasion

### Worry
Scores relate to subject's experience of worry in the past week, other than worry about physical Health.

*Score one for each of:*
- Symptom present on 4 or more days
- Has been worrying too much in view of circumstances
- Symptom has been very unpleasant
- Symptom lasted over three hours in total on any day

### Depression
Applies to subjects who felt sad, miserable or depressed or unable to enjoy or take an interest in things as much as usual, in the past week. Scores relate to the subject's experience in the past week.
*Score one for each of:*
- Unable to enjoy or take an interest in things as much as usual
- Symptom present on four days or more
- Symptom lasted for more than 3 hours in total on any day
- When sad, miserable or depressed subject did not become happier when something nice happened, or when in company

### Depressive ideas
Applies to subjects who had a score of 1 for depression. Scores relate to experience in the past week.
*Score one for each of:*
- Felt guilty or blamed him/herself when things went wrong when it had not been his/her fault
- Felt not as good as other people
- Felt hopeless
- Felt that life isn't worth living
- Thought of killing him/herself

### Anxiety
Scores relate to feeling generally anxious, nervous or tense in the past week. These feelings were not the result of a phobia.
*Score one for each of:*
- Symptom present on four or more days
- Symptom had been very unpleasant
- When anxious, nervous or tense, had one or more of following symptoms:
    heart racing or pounding
    hands sweating or shaking
    feeling dizzy
    difficulty getting breath
    butterflies in stomach
    dry mouth
    nausea or feeling as though he/she wanted to vomit

- Symptom present for more than three hours in total on any one day

## Obsessions

Scores relate to the subject's experience of having repetitive unpleasant thoughts or ideas in the past week.

*Score one for each of:*
- Symptom present on four or more days
- Tried to stop thinking any of these thoughts
- Became upset or annoyed when had these thoughts
- Longest episode of the symptom was ¼ hour or longer

## Concentration and forgetfulness

Scores relate to the subject's experience of concentration problems and forgetfulness in the past week.

*Score one for each of:*
- Symptoms present for four days or more
- Could not always concentrate on a TV programme, read a newspaper article or talk to someone without mind wandering
- Problems with concentration stopped subject from getting on with things he/she used to do or would have liked to do
- Forgot something important

## Somatic symptoms

Scores relate to the subject's experience in the past week of any ache, pain or discomfort which was brought on or made worse by feeling low, anxious or stressed.

*Score one for each of:*
- Symptom present for four days or more
- Symptom lasted more than 3 hours on any day
- Symptom had been very unpleasant
- Symptom bothered subject when doing something interesting

## Compulsions

Scores relate to the subject's experience of doing things over again when subject had already done them in the past week.

*Score one for each of:*
- Symptom present on four or more days
- Subject tried to stop repeating behaviour
- Symptom made subject upset or annoyed with him/herself
- Repeated behaviour three or more times when it had already been done

## Phobias

Scores relate to subject's experience of phobias or avoidance in the past week

*Score one for each of:*
- Felt nervous/anxious about a situation or thing four or more times
- On occasions when felt anxious, nervous or tense, had one or more of following symptoms:
  heart racing or pounding
  hands sweating or shaking
  feeling dizzy
  difficulty getting breath
  butterflies in stomach
  dry mouth
  nausea or feeling as though he/she wanted to vomit
- Avoided situation or thing at least once because it would have made subject anxious, nervous or tense

## Worry about physical health

Scores relate to experience of the symptom in the past week.

*Score one for each of:*
- Symptom present on four days or more
- Subject felt he/she had been worrying too much in view of actual health
- Symptom had been very unpleasant
- Subject could not be distracted by doing something else

## Panic

Applies to subjects who felt anxious, nervous or tense in the past week and the scores relate to the resultant feelings of panic, or of collapsing and losing control in the past week.

*Score one for each of:*
- Symptom experienced once
- Symptom experienced more than once
- Symptom had been very unpleasant or unbearable
- An episode lasted longer than 10 minutes

# B.2 Algorithms to produce ICD-10 psychiatric disorders

The mental disorders reported in Chapter 6 were produced from the CIS-R schedule which is described in Chapter 2 and reproduced in Appendix C. The production of the 6 categories of disorder shown in these tables occurred in 3 stages: first, the informants' responses to the CIS-R were used to produce specific ICD-10 diagnoses of neurosis.

This was done by applying the algorithms described below. Second, these specific neurotic disorders plus psychosis were arranged hierarchically and the 'highest' disorder assumed precedence. The actual precedence rules are described below. Finally, the range of ICD-10 diagnoses were grouped together to produce categories used in the calculation of prevalence.

It should be noted that as a result of the hierarchical coding described above, the diagnoses of the 6 neurotic disorders and the category of functional psychosis are exclusive: an individual included in the prevalence rates for one neurotic or psychotic disorder is not included in calculation of the rate for any other neurotic or psychotic disorder.

## Algorithms for production of ICD-10 diagnoses of neurosis from the CIS-R ('scores' refer to CIS-R scores)

### F32.00 Mild depressive episode without somatic symptoms

1. Symptom duration ≥ 2 weeks

2. *Two or more from:*

   - depressed mood
   - loss of interest
   - fatigue

3. *Two or three from:*

   - reduced concentration
   - reduced self-esteem
   - ideas of guilt
   - pessimism about future
   - suicidal ideas or acts
   - disturbed sleep
   - diminished appetite

4. Social impairment

5. *Fewer than four from:*

   - lack of normal pleasure /interest
   - loss of normal emotional reactivity
   - a.m. waking ≥ 2 hours early
   - loss of libido
   - diurnal variation in mood
   - diminished appetite
   - loss of ≥ 5% body weight
   - psychomotor agitation
   - psychomotor retardation

### F32.01 Mild depressive episode with somatic symptoms

1. Symptom duration ≥ 2 weeks

2. *Two or more from:*

   - depressed mood
   - loss of interest
   - fatigue

3. *Two or three from:*

   - reduced concentration
   - reduced self-esteem
   - ideas of guilt
   - pessimism about future
   - suicidal ideas or acts
   - disturbed sleep
   - diminished appetite

4. Social impairment

5. *Four or more from:*

   - lack of normal pleasure /interest
   - loss of normal emotional reactivity
   - a.m. waking ≥ 2 hours early
   - loss of libido
   - diurnal variation in mood
   - diminished appetite
   - loss of 5% body weight
   - psychomotor agitation
   - psychomotor retardation

### F32.10 Moderate depressive episode without somatic symptoms

1. Symptom duration ≥2 weeks

2. *Two or more* from:

   - depressed mood
   - loss of interest
   - fatigue

3. *Four or more* from:

   - reduced concentration
   - reduced self-esteem
   - ideas of guilt
   - pessimism about future
   - suicidal ideas or acts
   - disturbed sleep
   - diminished appetite

4. Social impairment

5. *Fewer than four* from:

   - lack of normal pleasure/interest
   - loss of normal emotional reactivity
   - a.m. waking ≥ 2 hours early
   - loss of libido
   - diurnal variation in mood
   - diminished appetite
   - loss of ≥ 5% body weight
   - psychomotor agitation
   - psychomotor retardation

**F32.11 Moderate depressive episode with somatic symptoms**

1. Symptom duration ≥2 weeks

2. *Two or more* from:

   - depressed mood
   - loss of interest
   - fatigue

3. *Four or more* from:

   - reduced concentration
   - reduced self-esteem
   - ideas of guilt
   - pessimism about future
   - suicidal ideas or acts
   - disturbed sleep
   - diminished appetite

4. Social impairment

5. *Four or more* from:

   - lack of normal pleasure /interest
   - loss of normal emotional reactivity
   - a.m. waking ≥2 hours early
   - loss of libido
   - diurnal variation in mood
   - diminished appetite
   - loss of ≥ 5% body weight
   - psychomotor agitation
   - psychomotor retardation

**F32.2 Severe depressive episode**

1. *All three* from:

   - depressed mood
   - loss of interest
   - fatigue

2. *Four or more* from:

   - reduced concentration
   - reduced self-esteem
   - ideas of guilt
   - pessimism about future
   - suicidal ideas or acts
   - disturbed sleep
   - diminished appetite

3. Social impairment

4. *Four or more* from:

   - lack of normal pleasure /interest
   - loss of normal emotional reactivity
   - a.m. waking ≥ 2 hours early
   - loss of libido
   - diurnal variation in mood
   - diminished appetite
   - loss of ≥ 5% body weight
   - psychomotor agitation
   - psychomotor retardation

**F40.00 Agoraphobia without panic disorder**

1. Fear of open spaces and related aspects: crowds, distance from home, travelling alone
2. Social impairment
3. Avoidant behaviour must be prominent feature
4. Overall phobia score ≥ 2
5. No panic attacks

**F40.01 Agoraphobia with panic disorder**

1. Fear of open spaces and related aspects: crowds, distance from home, travelling alone
2. Social impairment
3. Avoidant behaviour must be prominent feature
4. Overall phobia score ≥ 2
5. Panic disorder (overall panic score ≥ 2)

**F40.1 Social phobias**

1. Fear of scrutiny by other people: eating or speaking in public etc.
2. Social impairment
3. Avoidant behaviour must be prominent feature
4. Overall phobia score ≥ 2

**F40.2 Specific (isolated) phobias**

1. Fear of specific situations or things, e.g. animals, insects, heights, blood, flying, etc.
2. Social impairment
3. Avoidant behaviour must be prominent feature
4. Overall phobia score ≥ 2

### F41.0  Panic disorder
1.　　Criteria for phobic disorders not met
2.　　Recent panic attacks
3.　　Anxiety-free between attacks
4.　　Overall panic score $\geq 2$

### F41.1  Generalised Anxiety  Disorder
1.　　Duration $\geq 6$ months
2.　　Free-floating anxiety
3.　　Autonomic overactivity
4.　　Overall anxiety score $\geq 2$

### F41.2  Mixed anxiety and depressive disorder
1. (Sum of scores for each CIS-R section) $\geq 12$
2. Criteria for other categories not met

### F42  Obsessive-Compulsive Disorder
1. Duration $\geq 2$ weeks
2. At least one act/thought resisted
3. Social impairment
4. Overall scores:
　　obsession score=4, or
　　compulsion score=4, or
　　obsession+compulsion scores $\geq 6$

## Hierarchical organisation of psychiatric disorders

The following rules (see table below)  were used to allocate individuals who received more than one diagnosis of neurosis to the appropriate category.

## Grouping neurotic and psychotic disorders into broad categories

The final step was to group some of the diagnoses into broad diagnostic categories prior to analysis.

### Depressive episode
F32.00 and F32.01 were grouped to produce mild depressive episode (i.e. with or without somatic symptoms).  F32.10 and F32.11 were similarly grouped to produce moderate depressive episode. Mild depressive episode, moderate depressive episode and Severe depressive episode (F32.2) were then combined to produce the final category of depressive episode.

### Phobias
The ICD-10 phobic diagnoses F40.00, F40.01, F40.1 and F40.2, were combined into one category of phobia.

This produced six categories of neurosis  for analysis:
　　Mixed anxiety and depressive disorder
　　Generalised Anxiety Disorder
　　Depressive episode
　　All phobias
　　Obsessive Compulsive Disorder
　　Panic disorder

| Disorder 1 | Disorder 2 | Priority |
| --- | --- | --- |
| Depressive episode (any severity) | Phobia | Depressive episode  (any severity) |
| Depressive episode  (mild) | OCD | OCD |
| Depressive episode (moderate) | OCD | Depressive episode (moderate) |
| Depressive episode (severe) | OCD | Depressive episode  (severe) |
| Depressive episode (mild) | Panic disorder | Panic disorder |
| Depressive episode  (moderate) | Panic disorder | Depressive episode  (moderate) |
| Depressive episode (any severity) | GAD | Depressive episode (any severity) |
| Phobia (any) | OCD | OCD |
| Agoraphobia | GAD | Agoraphobia |
| Social phobia | GAD | Social phobia |
| Specific phobia | GAD | GAD |
| Panic disorder | OCD | Panic disorder |
| OCD | GAD | OCD |
| Panic disorder | GAD | Panic disorder |

GAD = Generalised Anxiety Disorder;  OCD = Obsessive– Compulsive Disorder

# B3 Non-neurotic disorders

All psychiatric disorders with the exception of neuroses were assessed from self-reports by patients or their staff. Sometimes residents did not use medical terms to describe their conditions: how their answers were interpreted into ICD-10 diagnostic categories is shown below:

## Primary diagnosis (based on ICD-10)

### F00 - F09  Organic Mental Disorders
Dementia
Alzheimer's Disease

### F10 - F19  Mental and behavioural disorders due to psychoactive substance use
Alcohol/heavy drinker
Opium
Cannabis
Sedatives
Cocaine
Stimulants
Hallucinogens
Tobacco
Volatile solvents
Any mixture of above

### F20 - F29  Schizophrenia, schizotypal and delusional disorders
Catatonic schizophrenia
Chronic schizophrenia
Hebephrenic schizophrenia
High schizophrenia
Mild schizophrenia
Paranoid schizophrenia
Schizophrenia
Simple schizophrenia

Auditory hallucinations
Hallucinations
Hearing voices
Mild psychosis
Psychosis
Psychotic tendencies
Schizoaffective disorder
Schizophrenic affective disorder
Voices

### F30 - F39  Mood (affective) disorders (excluding depressive episode)
Mania
Hyperactive
Hypomania
Mania
Manic depressive disorder
Bipolar affective disorder
Manic depression
Manic depressive psychosis
Moods
Mood swings

### F50 - F59  Behavioural syndromes associated with physiological disturbance and physical factors
Anorexia nervosa
Bulimia nervosa
Sleep disorders (non-organic), nightfrights
Sexual disorders (non-organic)
Other behavioural syndromes

### F60 - F69  Disorders of adult personality and behaviour
Habit and impulse disorders
Gender identity problems
Other personality disorders

### F70 - F79  Mental retardation
Mental handicap
Backward or slow

### F80 - F89  Disorders of psychological development

### F90 - F98  Behavioural and emotional disorders with onset usually occurring in childhood and adolescence

## Unspecified mental disorder
Mental illness
Mentally disturbed
Neuropathy

# Appendix C  Schedules A, B, D, E and accompanying documents

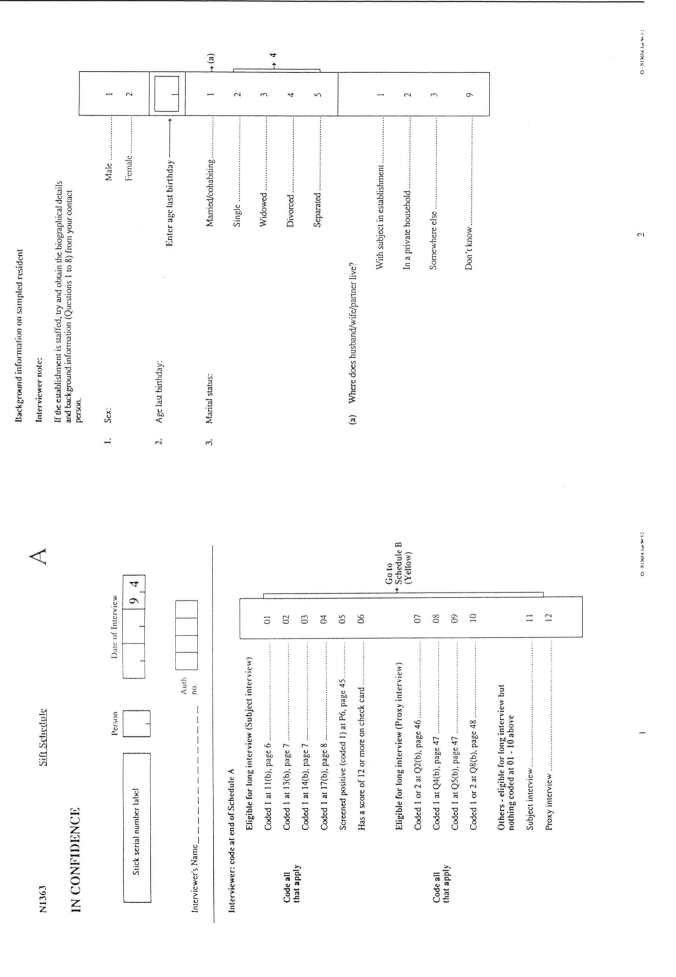

## Background information on sampled resident

**Interviewer note:**

If the establishment is staffed, try and obtain the biographical details and background information (Questions 1 to 8) from your contact person.

1. Sex:

| | |
|---|---|
| Male | 1 |
| Female | 2 |

2. Age last birthday:

Enter age last birthday ⟶ [ ]

3. Marital status:

| | |
|---|---|
| Married/cohabiting | 1 ⟶ (a) |
| Single | 2 |
| Widowed | 3 |
| Divorced | 4 ⟶ 4 |
| Separated | 5 |

(a) Where does husband/wife/partner live?

| | |
|---|---|
| With subject in establishment | 1 |
| In a private household | 2 |
| Somewhere else | 3 |
| Don't know | 9 |

2

---

N1363    Sift Schedule    A

## IN CONFIDENCE

Stick serial number label

Person [ ]    Date of Interview [ ][ ] 9 4

Auth no. _ _ _ _ _

Interviewer's Name _ _ _ _ _ _ _ _ _ _ _

**Interviewer: code at end of Schedule A**

**Eligible for long interview (Subject interview)**

| | |
|---|---|
| Coded 1 at 11(b), page 6 | 01 |
| Coded 1 at 13(b), page 7 | 02 |
| Coded 1 at 14(b), page 7 | 03 |
| Coded 1 at 17(b), page 8 | 04 |
| Screened positive (coded 1) at P6, page 45 | 05 |
| Has a score of 12 or more on check card | 06 |

**Eligible for long interview (Proxy interview)**

| | |
|---|---|
| Coded 1 or 2 at Q2(b), page 46 | 07 |
| Coded 1 at Q4(b), page 47 | 08 |
| Coded 1 at Q5(b), page 47 | 09 |
| Coded 1 or 2 at Q8(b), page 48 | 10 |

**Others - eligible for long interview but nothing coded at 01 - 10 above**

| | |
|---|---|
| Subject interview | 11 |
| Proxy interview | 12 |

**Code all that apply**

Go to Schedule B (Yellow)

1

5. How long has (SUBJECT) been at this (ESTABLISHMENT)?

Enter number of years →

or, if less than 1 year

Enter number of months
(less than 1 month = 00) →

If subject is in
hospital code
present episode

6. Where was (SUBJECT) living before coming here?

In a private household ......... 1

In (another) hospital, clinic
or nursing home ......... 2

In (another) residential home ......... 3

In supported accommodation
or group home ......... 4

Other (specify) ......... 5

Don't know ......... 9

4

O- N1363A Jan '94 V2

4 To which ethnic group does (SUBJECT) belong to?

Show card 1

White ......... 1

Black - Caribbean ......... 2

Black - African ......... 3

Black - Other ......... 4

Indian ......... 5

Pakistani ......... 6

Bangladeshi ......... 7

Chinese ......... 8

None of these ......... 9

3

O- N1363A Jan '94 V2

41

DNA: Interviewing subject ............... 1 → 9

**7** Is a move planned for (SUBJECT) in the next 12 months?

Yes ............... 1 → 8
No ............... 2 → 9
Don't know ............... 3 → 9

**8** Where would (SUBJECT) be moving to?

To a private household ............... 1
To (another) hospital, clinic or nursing home ............... 2
To (another) residential home ............... 3
To supported accommodation or group home ............... 4
Other (specify) ............... 5

**9** Interviewer check

Interview to continue with subject ............... 1 → See 10
Interview to continue with proxy ............... 2 → Section Q page 46

General health

**10** [*] How is your health in general? Would you say it was. . .

very good ............... 1
good ............... 2
fair ............... 3
bad ............... 4
or very bad? ............... 5

Running prompt

**11** [*] Do you have any long-standing illness, disability or infirmity? By long-standing I mean anything that has troubled you over a period of time or that is likely to affect you over a period of time?

Yes ............... 1 → (a)
No ............... 2 → 12

(a) What is the matter with you?

> **Try and obtain a medical diagnosis or establish main symptoms**

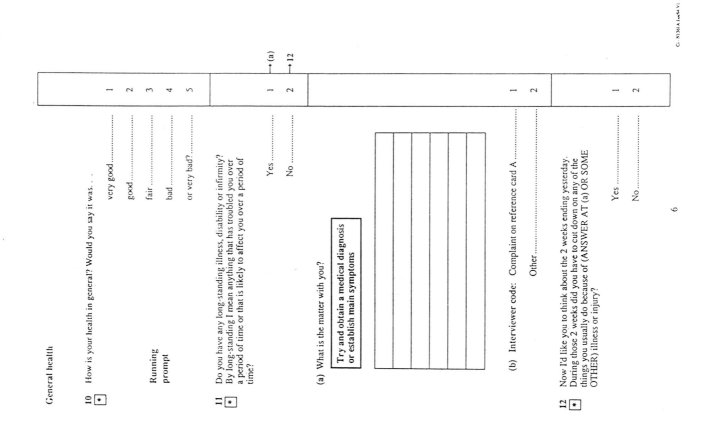

(b) Interviewer code: Complaint on reference card A ............... 1
Other ............... 2

**12** [*] Now I'd like you to think about the 2 weeks ending yesterday. During those 2 weeks did you have to cut down on any of the things you usually do because of (ANSWER AT (a) OR SOME OTHER) illness or injury?

Yes ............... 1
No ............... 2

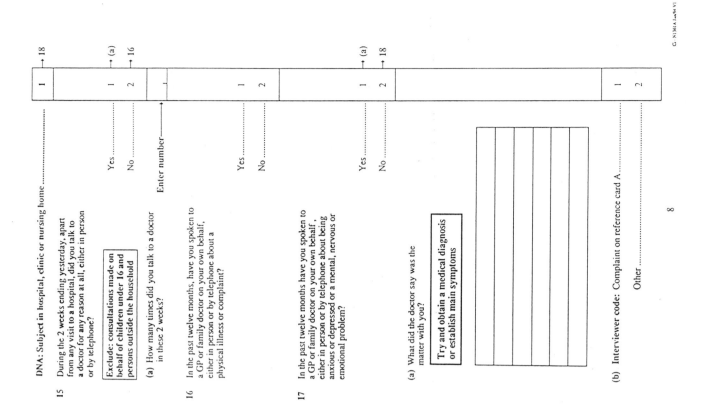

DNA: Subject in hospital, clinic or nursing home ................ → 18

15 During the 2 weeks ending yesterday, apart from any visit to a hospital, did you talk to a doctor for any reason at all, either in person or by telephone?

Exclude: consultations made on behalf of children under 16 and persons outside the household

   Yes ........... 1 → (a)
   No ........... 2 → 16

(a) How many times did you talk to a doctor in these 2 weeks?    Enter number ____

16 In the past twelve months, have you spoken to a GP or family doctor on your own behalf, either in person or by telephone about a physical illness or complaint?

   Yes ........... 1
   No ........... 2

17 In the past twelve months have you spoken to a GP or family doctor on your own behalf, either in person or by telephone about being anxious or depressed or a mental, nervous or emotional problem?

   Yes ........... 1 → (a)
   No ........... 2 → 18

(a) What did the doctor say was the matter with you?

Try and obtain a medical diagnosis or establish main symptoms

(b) Interviewer code:   Complaint on reference card A ........... 1

   Other ........... 2

8

G: N361A1a94 V1

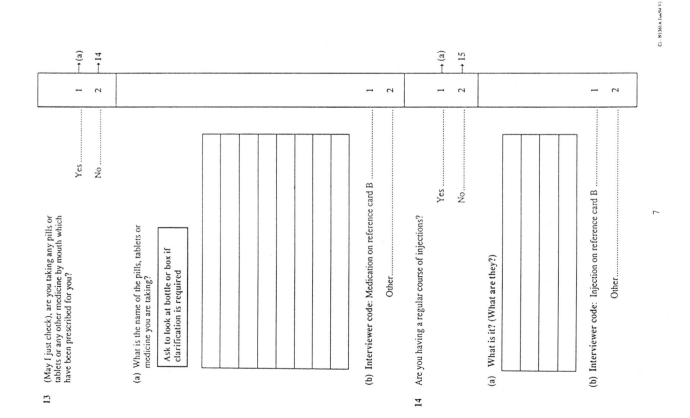

13 (May I just check), are you taking any pills or tablets or any other medicine by mouth which have been prescribed for you?

   Yes ........... 1 → (a)
   No ........... 2 → 14

(a) What is the name of the pills, tablets or medicine you are taking?

Ask to look at bottle or box if clarification is required

(b) Interviewer code:   Medication on reference card B ........... 1

   Other ........... 2

14 Are you having a regular course of injections?

   Yes ........... 1 → (a)
   No ........... 2 → 15

(a) What is it? (What are they?)

(b) Interviewer code:   Injection on reference card B ........... 1

   Other ........... 2

7

G: N361A1a94 V1

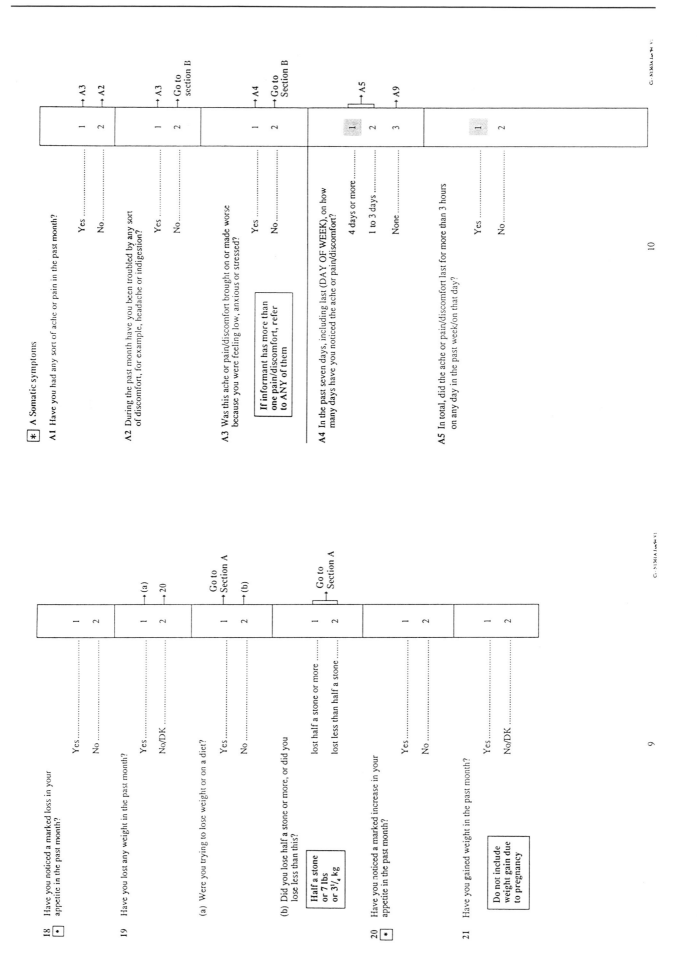

---

**18** [*] Have you noticed a marked loss in your appetite in the past month?

Yes ................................. 1

No ................................. 2

**19** Have you lost any weight in the past month?

Yes ................................. 1 → (a)

No/DK ................................. 2 → 20

(a) Were you trying to lose weight or on a diet?

Yes ................................. 1 → Go to Section A

No ................................. 2 → (b)

(b) Did you lose half a stone or more, or did you lose less than this?

lost half a stone or more ................................. 1 → Go to Section A

lost less than half a stone ................................. 2

| Half a stone or 7 lbs or 3¼ kg |

**20** [*] Have you noticed a marked increase in your appetite in the past month?

Yes ................................. 1

No ................................. 2

**21** Have you gained weight in the past month?

Yes ................................. 1

No/DK ................................. 2

| Do not include weight gain due to pregnancy |

9

---

[*] **A Somatic symptoms**

**A1** Have you had any sort of ache or pain in the past month?

Yes ................................. 1 → A3

No ................................. 2 → A2

**A2** During the past month have you been troubled by any sort of discomfort, for example, headache or indigestion?

Yes ................................. 1 → A3

No ................................. 2 → Go to section B

**A3** Was this ache or pain/discomfort brought on or made worse because you were feeling low, anxious or stressed?

Yes ................................. 1 → A4

No ................................. 2 → Go to Section B

| If informant has more than one pain/discomfort, refer to ANY of them |

**A4** In the past seven days, including last (DAY OF WEEK), on how many days have you noticed the ache or pain/discomfort?

4 days or more ................................. 1 → A5

1 to 3 days ................................. 2

None ................................. 3 → A9

**A5** In total, did the ache or pain/discomfort last for more than 3 hours on any day in the past week/on that day?

Yes ................................. 1

No ................................. 2

10

## A6–A9

A6  In the past week, has the ache or pain/discomfort been

**Running prompt**

very unpleasant .......... 1

a little unpleasant .......... 2

or not unpleasant? .......... 3

A7  Has the ache or pain/discomfort bothered you when you were doing something interesting in the past week?

Yes .......... 1

No/has not done anything interesting .......... 2

A8  How long have you been feeling this ache or pain/discomfort as you have just described?

Show card 2

less than 2 weeks .......... 1

2 weeks but less than 6 months .......... 2

6 months but less than 1 year .......... 3

1 year but less than 2 years .......... 4

2 years or more .......... 5

A9  Interviewer check:

Sum codes which you have ringed in the shaded boxes at A4, A5, A6 and A7.

Ring '0' if sum of codes is zero .......... 0

or

enter score ————

→ Insert score on check card, then go to section B

11

---

## * B Fatigue

B1  Have you noticed that you've been getting tired in the past month?

Yes .......... 1 → B3

No .......... 2 → B2

B2  During the past month, have you felt you've been lacking in energy?

Yes .......... 1 → B3

No .......... 2 → Go to section C

B3  Do you know why you have been feeling tired/lacking in energy?

Yes .......... 1 → (a)

No .......... 2 → B4

(a)  What is the main reason? Can you choose from this card?

Show card 3

Code one only

Problems with sleep .......... 1

Medication .......... 2

Physical illness .......... 3  → B4

Working too hard (inc. housework, looking after baby) .......... 4

Stress, worry or other psychological reason .......... 5

Physical exercise .......... 6 → Go to section C

Other .......... 7 → B4

B4  In the past seven days, including last (DAY OF WEEK) on how many days have you felt tired/lacking in energy?

4 days or more .......... 1 → B5

1 to 3 days .......... 2

None .......... 3 → B10

B5  Have you felt tired/lacking in energy for more than 3 hours in total on any day in the past week?

Yes .......... 1

No .......... 2

Exclude time spent sleeping

12

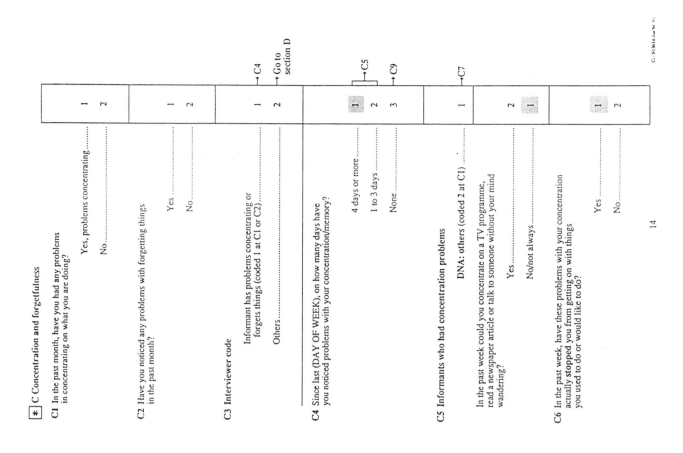

* **C  Concentration and forgetfulness**

C1  In the past month, have you had any problems in concentrating on what you are doing?
  Yes, problems concentrating .......... 1
  No .......... 2

C2  Have you noticed any problems with forgetting things in the past month?
  Yes .......... 1
  No .......... 2

C3  Interviewer code
  Informant has problems concentrating or forgets things (coded 1 at C1 or C2) .......... 1 → C4
  Others .......... 2 → Go to section D

C4  Since last (DAY OF WEEK), on how many days have you noticed problems with your concentration/memory?
  4 days or more .......... 1 ┐
  1 to 3 days .......... 2 ┘ → C5
  None .......... 3 → C9

C5  Informants who had concentration problems
  In the past week could you concentrate on a TV programme, read a newspaper article or talk to someone without your mind wandering?
  DNA: others (coded 2 at C1) .......... 1 → C7
  Yes .......... 2
  No/not always .......... 1

C6  In the past week, have these problems with your concentration actually stopped you from getting on with things you used to do or would like to do?
  Yes .......... 1
  No .......... 2

14

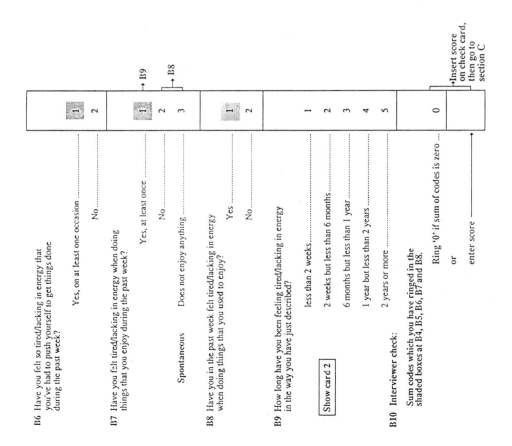

B6  Have you felt so tired/lacking in energy that you've had to push yourself to get things done during the past week?
  Yes, on at least one occasion .......... 1
  No .......... 2

B7  Have you felt tired/lacking in energy when doing things that you enjoy during the past week?
  Yes, at least once .......... 1 → B9
  No .......... 2
  Spontaneous    Does not enjoy anything .......... 3 → B8

B8  Have you in the past week felt tired/lacking in energy when doing things that you used to enjoy?
  Yes .......... 1
  No .......... 2

B9  How long have you been feeling tired/lacking in energy in the way you have just described?
  less than 2 weeks .......... 1
  2 weeks but less than 6 months .......... 2
  6 months but less than 1 year .......... 3
  1 year but less than 2 years .......... 4
  2 years or more .......... 5

Show card 2

B10  Interviewer check:
  Sum codes which you have ringed in the shaded boxes at B4, B5, B6, B7 and B8.
  Ring '0' if sum of codes is zero ... 0
  or
  enter score ___ → Insert score on check card, then go to section C

13

[*] **D Sleep problems**

**D1** In the past month, have you been having problems with trying to get to sleep or with getting back to sleep if you woke up or were woken up?

Yes ......... 1 → D3
No .......... 2 → D2

**D2** Has sleeping more than you usually do been a problem for you in the past month?

Yes ......... 1 → D3
No .......... 2 → Go to section E

**D3** On how many of the past seven nights did you have problems with your sleep?

4 nights or more ......... 1 ⎫
1 to 3 nights ............. 2 ⎬ → D4
None ...................... 3 → D11

**D4** Do you know why you are having problems with your sleep?

Yes ......... 1 → (a)
No .......... 2 → D5

(a) Can you look at this card and tell me the main reason for these problems?

Show card 4

Code one only

Noise ......................................... 1
Shift work/too busy to sleep ................ 2
Illness/discomfort .......................... 3
Worry/thinking .............................. 4
Needing to go to the toilet ................. 5
Having to do something (e.g. look after baby) . 6
Tired ....................................... 7
Medication .................................. 8
Other ....................................... 9

16

**C7 Informants who had memory problems**

DNA: others (coded 2 at C2) ......... 1 → C8

(Earlier you said you have been forgetting things.) Have you forgotten anything important in the past seven days?

Yes ......... 1
No .......... 2

**C8** How long have you been having the problems with your concentration/memory as you have described?

Show card 2

Less than 2 weeks ......................... 1
2 weeks but less than 6 months ............ 2
6 months but less than 1 year ............. 3
1 year but less than 2 years .............. 4
2 years or more ........................... 5

**C9 Interviewer check:**

Sum codes which you have ringed in the shaded boxes at C4, C5, C6 and C7.

Ring '0' if sum of codes is zero ... 0 → Insert score on check card, then go to section D

or

enter score ——————

15

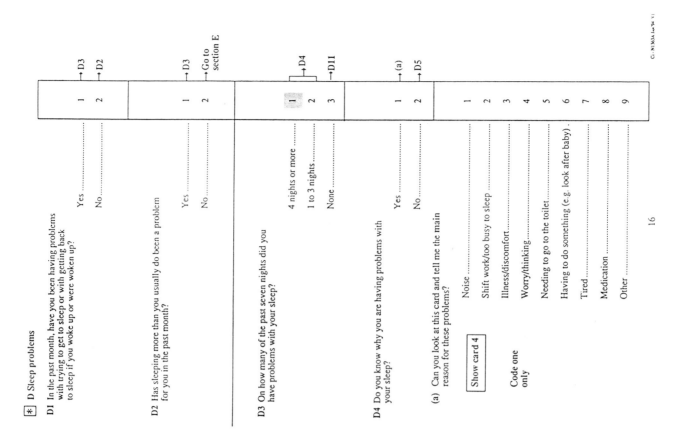

47

**D10** How long have you had these problems with your sleep as you have described?

Show card 2

| | |
|---|---|
| less than 2 weeks | 1 |
| 2 weeks but less than 6 months | 2 |
| 6 months but less than 1 year | 3 |
| 1 year but less than 2 years | 4 |
| 2 years or more | 5 |

**D11 Interviewer check:**

Sum codes which you have ringed in the shaded boxes at D3, D5, D6, D8 and D9.

| | |
|---|---|
| Ring '0' if sum of codes is zero (or if coded 3 at D5 or D8) | 0 |
| or | |
| enter score | → Insert score on Check card, then go to section E |

18

---

**D5 Informants who had problems trying to get (back) to sleep**

| | | |
|---|---|---|
| DNA : others (coded 2 at D1) | 1 | → D8 |

Thinking about the night you had the least sleep in the past week, how long did you spend trying to get to sleep? (If you woke up or were woken up I want you to allow a quarter of an hour to get back to sleep).

Only include time spent trying to get to sleep.

| | | |
|---|---|---|
| Less than 1/4 hr | 3 | → Go to D11 and code '0' |
| At least 1/4 hr but less than 1 hr | 1 | → D7 |
| At least 1 hr but less than 3 hrs | 2 | |
| 3 hrs or more | 2 | → D6 |

**D6** In the past week, on how many nights did you spend 3 or more hours trying to get to sleep?

| | |
|---|---|
| 4 nights or more | 1 |
| 1 to 3 nights | 2 |
| None | 3 |

**D7** Do you wake more than two hours earlier than you need to and then find you can't get back to sleep?

| | | |
|---|---|---|
| Yes | 1 | → D10 |
| No | 2 | |

**D8 Informants who slept more than usual**

Thinking about the night you slept the longest in the past week, how much longer did you sleep compared with how long you normally sleep for?

| | | |
|---|---|---|
| Less than 1/4 hr | 3 | → Go to D11 and code '0' |
| At least 1/4 hr but less than 1 hr | 1 | → D10 |
| At least 1 hr but less than 3 hrs | 2 | |
| 3 hrs or more | 2 | → D9 |

**D9** In the past week, on how many nights did you sleep for more than 3 hours longer than you usually do?

| | |
|---|---|
| 4 nights or more | 1 |
| 1 to 3 nights | 2 |
| None | 3 |

17

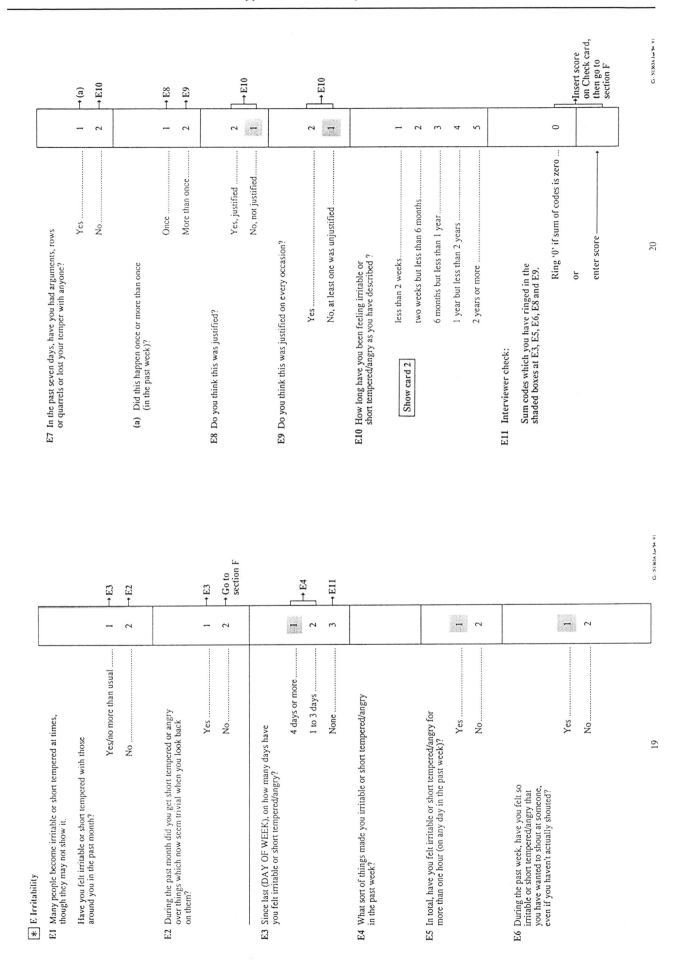

* **E Irritability**

**E1** Many people become irritable or short tempered at times, though they may not show it.

Have you felt irritable or short tempered with those around you in the past month?

| | | |
|---|---|---|
| Yes/no more than usual | 1 | → E3 |
| No | 2 | → E2 |

**E2** During the past month did you get short tempered or angry over things which now seem trivial when you look back on them?

| | | |
|---|---|---|
| Yes | 1 | → E3 |
| No | 2 | → Go to section F |

**E3** Since last (DAY OF WEEK), on how many days have you felt irritable or short tempered/angry?

| | | |
|---|---|---|
| 4 days or more | 1 | → E4 |
| 1 to 3 days | 2 | |
| None | 3 | → E11 |

**E4** What sort of things made you irritable or short tempered/angry in the past week?

**E5** In total, have you felt irritable or short tempered/angry for more than one hour (on any day in the past week)?

| | |
|---|---|
| Yes | 1 |
| No | 2 |

**E6** During the past week, have you felt so irritable or short tempered/angry that you have wanted to shout at someone, even if you haven't actually shouted?

| | |
|---|---|
| Yes | 1 |
| No | 2 |

19

**E7** In the past seven days, have you had arguments, rows or quarrels or lost your temper with anyone?

| | | |
|---|---|---|
| Yes | 1 | → (a) |
| No | 2 | → E10 |

(a) Did this happen once or more than once (in the past week)?

| | | |
|---|---|---|
| Once | 1 | → E8 |
| More than once | 2 | → E9 |

**E8** Do you think this was justified?

| | | |
|---|---|---|
| Yes, justified | 2 | |
| No, not justified | 1 | → E10 |

**E9** Do you think this was justified on every occasion?

| | | |
|---|---|---|
| Yes | 2 | |
| No, at least one was unjustified | 1 | → E10 |

**E10** How long have you been feeling irritable or short tempered/angry as you have described?

Show card 2

| | |
|---|---|
| less than 2 weeks | 1 |
| two weeks but less than 6 months | 2 |
| 6 months but less than 1 year | 3 |
| 1 year but less than 2 years | 4 |
| 2 years or more | 5 |

**E11** Interviewer check:
Sum codes which you have ringed in the shaded boxes at E3, E5, E6, E8 and E9.

| | |
|---|---|
| Ring '0' if sum of codes is zero | 0 |
| or | |
| enter score → | |

→ Insert score on Check card, then go to section F

20

49

## F Worry about physical health

**F1** Many people get concerned about their physical health. In the past month, have you been at all worried about your physical health?

| Include women who are worried about their pregnancy |
|---|

Yes, worried .......... 1 → F3
No/concerned .......... 2 → F2

**F2** Informants who have no problems with physical health

DNA : has a physical health problem shown at 11a <u>page 6</u> .......... 1 → Go to section G

During the past month, did you find yourself worrying that you might have a serious physical illness?

Yes .......... 1 → F3
No .......... 2 → Go to section G

**F3** Thinking about the past seven days, including last (DAY OF WEEK), on how many days have you found yourself worrying about your physical health/that you might have a serious physical illness?

4 days or more .......... 1
1 to 3 days .......... 2 → F4
None .......... 3 → F8

**F4** In your opinion, have you been worrying too much in view of your actual health?

Yes .......... 1
No .......... 2

**F5** In the past week, has this worrying been

Running prompt

very unpleasant .......... 1
a little unpleasant .......... 2
or not unpleasant? .......... 3

**F6** In the past week, have you been able to take your mind off your health worries at least once, by doing something else?

Yes .......... 2
No, could not be distracted once .......... 1

**F7** How long have you been worrying about your physical health in the way you have described?

| Show card 2 |
|---|

less than 2 weeks .......... 1
2 weeks but less than 6 months .......... 2
6 months but less than 1 year .......... 3
1 year but less than 2 years .......... 4
2 years or more .......... 5

**F8** Interviewer check:

Sum codes which you have ringed in the shaded boxes at F3, F4, F5 and F6.

Ring '0' if sum of codes is zero .......... 0
or
enter score →

→ Insert score on Check card, then go to section G

21

22

**•** **G Depression**

**G1** Almost everyone becomes sad, miserable or depressed at times.
Have you had a spell of feeling sad, miserable or depressed in the past month?

| | |
|---|---|
| Yes | 1 |
| No | 2 |

**G2** During the past month, have you been able to enjoy or take an interest in things as much as you usually do?

| | |
|---|---|
| Yes | 1 |
| No/no enjoyment or interest | 2 |

**G3** Interviewer check:

Code first that applies

| | | |
|---|---|---|
| Informant felt sad, miserable or depressed (coded 1 at G1) | 1 | → G4 |
| Informant unable to enjoy or take an interest (coded 2 at G2) | 2 | → G5 |
| Others | 3 | → Go to Section I, page 28 |

**G4** In the past week have you had a spell of feeling sad, miserable or depressed?

[Use informant's own words if possible]

| | | |
|---|---|---|
| Yes | 1 | → See G5 |
| No | 2 | |

**G5** Informants who were unable to enjoy or take an interest in things

In the past week have you been able to enjoy or take an interest in things as much as usual?

| | | |
|---|---|---|
| DNA: coded 1 at G2 | 1 | → See G6 |

[Use informant's own words if possible]

| | |
|---|---|
| Yes | 2 |
| No/no enjoyment or interest | 1 |

23

**G6** Informants who felt **sad, miserable or depressed or unable to enjoy or take an interest in things in the past week** (coded 1 at G4 or G5)

| | | |
|---|---|---|
| DNA: others | 1 | → Go to G11 |

Since last (DAY OF WEEK) on how many days have you felt sad, miserable or depressed/unable to enjoy or take an interest in things?

| | |
|---|---|
| 4 days or more | 1 |
| 2 to 3 days | 2 |
| 1 day | 3 |

**G7** Have you felt sad, miserable or depressed/unable to enjoy or take an interest in things for more than 3 hours in total (on any day in the past week)?

| | |
|---|---|
| Yes | 1 |
| No | 2 |

**G8 (a)** What sorts of things made you feel sad, miserable or depressed/unable to enjoy or take an interest in things in the past week? Can you choose from this card?

Ring code(s) in column (a).

[Show card 5]

| | (a) Code all that apply | (b) Code one only |
|---|---|---|
| Members of the family | 01 | 01 |
| Relationship with spouse/partner | 02 | 02 |
| Relationships with friends | 03 | 03 |
| Housing | 04 | 04 |
| Money/bills | 05 | 05 |
| Own physical health (inc. pregnancy) | 06 | 06 |
| Own mental health | 07 | 07 |
| Work or lack of work (inc. student) | 08 | 08 |
| Legal difficulties | 09 | 09 |
| Political issues/the news | 10 | 10 |
| Other | 11 | 11 |
| Don't know/no main thing | 99 | 99 |

**(b)**

| | | |
|---|---|---|
| DNA : Only one item coded at (a) | 1 | → G9 |

What was the main thing?
Ring code in column (b)

24

**• I1 Depressive Ideas**

**I1.1 Informants who scored 1 or more at section G, Depression**

DNA: Others (coded O or blank at G11) .............. 1 → Go to section I

*I would now like to ask you about when you have been feeling sad, miserable or depressed/unable to enjoy or take an interest in things. In the past week, was this worse in the morning or in the evening, or did this make no difference?*

| | | |
|---|---|---|
| Prompt as necessary | in the morning .......... | 1 |
| | in the evening .......... | 2 |
| | no difference/other ...... | 3 |

**H2** [Ask or use card 7]

*Many people find that feeling sad, miserable or depressed/unable to enjoy or take an interest in things can affect their interest in sex. Over the past month, do you think your interest in sex has*

| | | |
|---|---|---|
| Running prompt | increased .......... | 1 |
| | decreased .......... | 2 |
| | or has it stayed the same? ...... | 3 |
| Spontaneous | Not applicable .......... | 4 |

**H3** When you have felt sad, miserable or depressed/unable to enjoy or take an interest in things in the past seven days,

| | Yes | No |
|---|---|---|
| have you been so restless that you couldn't sit still? | 1 | 2 |
| *Individual prompt* have you been doing things more slowly, for example, walking more slowly? | 1 | 2 |
| have you been less talkative than normal? | 1 | 2 |

**H4** Now, thinking about the past seven days have you on at least one occasion felt guilty or blamed yourself when things went wrong when it hasn't been your fault?

| | |
|---|---|
| Yes, at least once .......... | 1 |
| No .......... | 2 |

**H5** During the past week, have you been feeling you are not as good as other people?

| | |
|---|---|
| Yes .......... | 1 |
| No .......... | 2 |

**H6** Have you felt hopeless at all during the past seven days, for instance about your future?

| | |
|---|---|
| Yes .......... | 1 |
| No .......... | 2 |

---

**G9** In the past week when you felt sad, miserable or depressed/unable to enjoy or take an interest in things, did you ever become happier when something nice happened, or when you were in company?

| | |
|---|---|
| Yes, at least once .......... | 2 |
| No .......... | 1 |

**G10** How long have you been feeling sad, miserable or depressed/unable to enjoy or take an interest in things as you have described?

[Show card 6]

| | |
|---|---|
| less than 2 weeks .......... | 1 |
| 2 weeks but less than 6 months .......... | 2 |
| 6 months but less than 1 year .......... | 3 |
| 1 year but less than 2 years .......... | 4 |
| 2 years or more .......... | 5 |

**G11 Interviewer check:**

Sum codes which you have ringed in the shaded boxes at G5, G6, G7 and G9.

| | |
|---|---|
| Ring '0' if sum of codes is zero ... | 0 |

or

enter score → Insert score on Check card, then go to section H

## • I Worry

**I1** (The next few questions are about worrying.)
In the past month, did you find yourself worrying more than you needed to about things?

| | | |
|---|---|---|
| Yes, worrying | 1 | → I3 |
| No/concerned | 2 | → I2 |

**I2** Have you had any worries at all in the past month?

| | | |
|---|---|---|
| Yes | 1 | → I3 |
| No | 2 | → Go to section J |

**I3 (a)** Can you look at this card and tell me what sorts of things you worried about in the past month?

Ring code(s) in column (a).

Show card 10

| | (a) Code all that apply | (b) Code one only |
|---|---|---|
| Members of the family | 01 | 01 |
| Relationship with spouse/partner | 02 | 02 |
| Relationships with friends | 03 | 03 |
| Housing | 04 | 04 |
| Money/bills | 05 | 05 |
| Own physical health (inc. pregnancy) | 06 | 06 |
| Own mental health | 07 | 07 |
| Work or lack of work (inc student) | 08 | 08 |
| Legal difficulties | 09 | 09 |
| Political issues/the news | 10 | 10 |
| Other | 11 | 11 |
| Don't know/no main thing | 99 | 99 |

DNA : Only one item coded at (a) ............ 1 → I4

**(b)** What was the main thing you worried about?
Ring code in column (b).

**I4** Interviewer check:

| | | |
|---|---|---|
| Informant worries about physical health (coded 06 at I3(a)) | 1 | See instruction below, then go to I5 |
| Others (not coded 06 at I3(a)) | 2 | → I6 |

Make a note on Check flap to go to section F to record this worry about physical health, if not already recorded.

28

---

**H7** Interviewer check

| | | |
|---|---|---|
| Informant felt guilty, not as good as others or hopeless (coded 1 at H4 or H5 or H6) | 1 | → H8 |
| Others (coded 2 at H4, H5 and H6) | 2 | → read H10 |

**H8** Ask or use card 8

In the past week have you felt that life isn't worth living?

| | | |
|---|---|---|
| Yes | 1 | → H9 |
| Spontaneous: Yes, but not in the past week | 2 | → read H10 |
| No | 3 | → read H10 |

**H9** Ask or use card 9

In the past week, have you thought of killing yourself?

| | | |
|---|---|---|
| Yes | 1 | → (a) |
| Spontaneous: Yes, but not in the past week | 2 | → read H10 |
| No | 3 | → read H10 |

**(a)** Have you talked to your doctor about these thoughts (of killing yourself)?

| | | |
|---|---|---|
| Yes | 1 | → read H10 |
| Spontaneous: No, but has talked to other people | 2 | → read (b) |
| No | 3 | → read H10 |

**(b)** (You have said that you are thinking about committing suicide.)
Since this is a very serious matter it is important that you talk to your doctor about these thoughts. → read H10

**H10** (Thank you for answering those questions on how you have been feeling. I would now like to ask you a few questions about worrying.)

**H11** Interviewer check:

Sum codes which you have ringed in the shaded boxes at H4, H5, H6, H8 and H9.

| | | |
|---|---|---|
| Ring '0' if sum of codes is zero | 0 | Insert score on Check card, then go to section I |

or

enter score _____

Maximum score on this section is 5

27

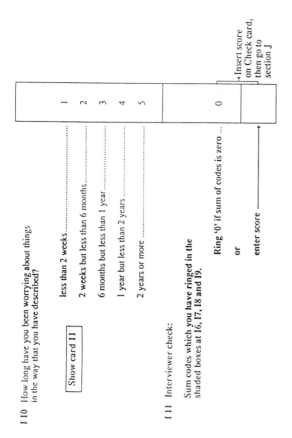

I 10  How long have you been worrying about things in the way that you have described?

Show card 11

| | |
|---|---|
| less than 2 weeks | 1 |
| 2 weeks but less than 6 months | 2 |
| 6 months but less than 1 year | 3 |
| 1 year but less than 2 years | 4 |
| 2 years or more | 5 |

I 11  Interviewer check:

Sum codes which you have ringed in the shaded boxes at I6, I7, I8 and I9.

**Ring '0' if sum of codes is zero** ... 0

or

enter score ────────→

→ Insert score on Check card, then go to section J

I 5  Interviewer check:

Informant **is only** worried about physical health (only code 06 is rung at I3(a)) ... 1 → Go to section J

Informant had other worries (I3(a) is multi-coded) ... 2 → read (a)

(a) For the next few questions, I want you to think about the worries you have had other than those about your physical health.

I 6  On how many of the past seven days have you been worrying about things (other than your physical health)?

| | | |
|---|---|---|
| 4 days or more | 1 | → I7 |
| 1 to 3 days | 2 | |
| None | 3 | → I11 |

I 7  In your opinion, have you been worrying too much in view of your circumstances?

| | |
|---|---|
| Yes | 1 |
| No | 2 |

**Refer to worries other than those about physical health**

I 8  In the past week, has this worrying been:

**Running prompt**

| | |
|---|---|
| very unpleasant | 1 |
| a little unpleasant | 2 |
| or not unpleasant? | 3 |

**Refer to worries other than those about physical health**

I 9  Have you worried for more than 3 hours in total on any one of the past seven days?

| | |
|---|---|
| Yes | 1 |
| No | 2 |

**Refer to worries other than those about physical health**

# J Anxiety

**J1** Have you been feeling anxious or nervous in the past month?

| | | |
|---|---|---|
| Yes, anxious or nervous | 1 | → J3 |
| No | 2 | → J2 |

**J2** In the past month, did you ever find your muscles felt tense or that you couldn't relax?

| | |
|---|---|
| Yes | 1 |
| No | 2 |

**J3** Some people have phobias; they get nervous or uncomfortable about specific things or situations when there is no real danger. For instance they may get nervous when speaking or eating in front of strangers, when they are far from home or in crowded rooms, or they may have a fear of heights. Others become nervous at the sight of things like blood or spiders.

In the past month have you felt anxious, nervous or tense about any specific things or situations when there was no real danger?

| | |
|---|---|
| Yes | 1 |
| No | 2 |

**J4 Interviewer check:**

| | | |
|---|---|---|
| Informant reports anxiety and also a phobia (coded 1 at J1 or J2, and coded 1 at J3) | 1 | → J5 |
| Informant reports only general anxiety (coded 1 at J1 or J2, and coded 2 at J3) | 2 | → J7 |
| Others (coded 2 at J1 and J2, and coded 1 or 2 at J3) | 3 | → Go to section K |

**J5** In the past month, when you felt anxious/nervous/tense, was this always brought on by the phobia about some specific situation or thing or did you sometimes feel generally anxious/nervous/tense?

| | | |
|---|---|---|
| Always brought on by phobia | 1 | → Go to section K |
| Sometimes felt generally anxious | 2 | → J6 |

31

**J6** The next questions are concerned with **general anxiety/nervousness/tension only.** I will ask you about the anxiety which is brought on by the phobia about specific things or situations later.

On how many of the past seven days have you felt **generally anxious/nervous/tense?**

| | | |
|---|---|---|
| 4 days or more | 1 | → J8 |
| 1 to 3 days | 2 | |
| None | 3 | → J12 |

**J7** On how many of the past seven days have you felt generally anxious/nervous/tense?

| | | |
|---|---|---|
| 4 days or more | 1 | → J8 |
| 1 to 3 days | 2 | |
| None | 3 | → J12 |

**J8** In the past week, has your anxiety/nervousness/tension been:

**Running prompt**

| | |
|---|---|
| very unpleasant | 1 |
| a little unpleasant | 2 |
| or not unpleasant? | 3 |

**J9** In the past week, when you've been anxious/nervous/tense, have you had any of the symptoms shown on this card?

| | | |
|---|---|---|
| Yes | 1 | → (a) |
| No | 2 | → J10 |

Show card 12

(a) Which of these symptoms did you have when you felt anxious/nervous/tense?

Code all that apply

| | |
|---|---|
| Heart racing or pounding | 1 |
| Hands sweating or shaking | 2 |
| Feeling dizzy | 3 |
| Difficulty getting your breath | 4 |
| Butterflies in stomach | 5 |
| Dry mouth | 6 |
| Nausea or feeling as though you wanted to vomit | 7 |

If informant had any of these symptoms, check J9 is coded 1, 'Yes'.

32

J10 Have you felt anxious/nervous/tense for more than 3 hours in total on any one of the past seven days?

Yes ............... 1
No ............... 2

J11 How long have you had these feelings of general anxiety/nervousness/tension as you described?

Show card 11

less than 2 weeks ............... 1
2 weeks but less than 6 months ............... 2
6 months but less than 1 year ............... 3
1 year but less than 2 years ............... 4
2 years or more ............... 5

J12 Interviewer check:

Sum codes which you have ringed in the shaded boxes at J6, J7, J8, J9 and J10.

Ring '0' if sum of codes is zero ... 0

or

enter score _____

→ Insert score on Check card, then go to section K

● K Phobias

K1 Interviewer check:

Informants who had phobic anxiety in the past month (coded 1 at J3) ............... 1 → K3(a)

Others ............... 2 → K2

K2 Sometimes people avoid a specific situation or thing, because they have a phobia about it. For instance, some people avoid eating in public or avoid going to busy places because it would make them feel nervous or anxious.

In the past month, have you avoided any situation or thing because it would have made you feel nervous or anxious, even though there was no real danger?

Yes ............... 1 → K3(b)
No ............... 2 → See section L

K3(a) Can you look at this card and tell me which of the situations or things listed made you the most anxious/nervous/tense in the past month? Ring code at (b), then go to K4

Show card 13

(b) Can you look at this card and tell me, which of these situations or things did you avoid the most in the past month?

Show card 13

Code one only

Crowds or public places, including travelling alone or being far from home ............... 1
Enclosed spaces ............... 2
Social situations, including eating or speaking in public, being watched or stared at ............... 3
The sight of blood or injury ............... 4
Any specific single cause including insects, spiders and heights ............... 5
Other (specify) ............... 6

K4 Informants who had phobic anxiety in past month

DNA: others (coded 2 at K1) ............... 1 → K7

In the past seven days, how many times have you felt nervous or anxious about (SITUATION/THING)?

4 times or more ............... 1 → K5
1 to 3 times ............... 2
None ............... 3 → K6

## L Panic

**L1 Informants who felt anxious in the past month**

| | | |
|---|---|---|
| DNA: Others (coded 3 at J4, page 31) | 1 | → Go to section M |

Thinking about the past month, did your anxiety or tension ever get so bad that you got in a panic, for instance make you feel that you might collapse or lose control unless you did something about it?

| | | |
|---|---|---|
| Yes | 1 | → L2 |
| No | 2 | → Go to section M |

**L2** How often has this happened in the past week?

| | | |
|---|---|---|
| Once | 1 | ⎤ → L3 |
| More than once | 2 | ⎦ |
| Not at all | 3 | → L8 |

**L3** In the past week, have these feelings of panic been:

**Running prompt**

| | |
|---|---|
| a little uncomfortable or unpleasant | 2 |
| or have they been very unpleasant or unbearable? | 1 |

**L4** Did this panic/the worst of these panics last for longer than 10 minutes?

| | |
|---|---|
| Yes | 1 |
| No | 2 |

**L5** Are you relatively free of anxiety between these panics?

| | |
|---|---|
| Yes | 1 |
| No | 2 |

36

---

**K5** In the past week, on those occasions when you felt anxious/nervous/tense did you have any of the symptoms on this card?

Show card 12

| | | |
|---|---|---|
| Yes | 1 | → (a) |
| No | 2 | → K6 |

**(a)** Which of these symptoms did you have when you felt anxious/nervous/tense?

Code all that apply

| | |
|---|---|
| Heart racing or pounding | 1 |
| Hands sweating or shaking | 2 |
| Feeling dizzy | 3 |
| Difficulty getting your breath | 4 |
| Butterflies in stomach | 5 |
| Dry mouth | 6 |
| Nausea or feeling as though you wanted to vomit | 7 |

If informant had any of these symptoms, check K5 is coded 1, 'Yes'.

**K6** In the past week, have you avoided any situation or thing because it would have made you feel anxious/nervous/tense even though there was no real danger?

| | | |
|---|---|---|
| Yes | 1 | → K7 |
| No | 2 | → K8 |

**K7** How many times have you avoided such situations or things in the past seven days?

| | | |
|---|---|---|
| 1 to 3 times | 1 | |
| 4 times or more | 2 | |
| None | 3 | → K9 |

**K8 Informants who had phobic anxiety/avoidance in the past week** (coded 1 or 2 at K4 or K7)

| | |
|---|---|
| DNA: others | 1 |

How long have you been having these feelings about these situations/things as you have just described?

Show card 14

| | |
|---|---|
| less than 2 weeks | 1 |
| 2 weeks but less than 6 months | 2 |
| 6 months but less than 1 year | 3 |
| 1 year but less than 2 years | 4 |
| 2 years or more | 5 |

**K9** Interviewer check:

Sum codes which you have ringed in the shaded boxes at K4, K5 and K7.

| | | |
|---|---|---|
| Ring '0' if sum of codes is zero | 0 | Insert score on Check card, then see section L |
| or | | |
| enter score | | |

35

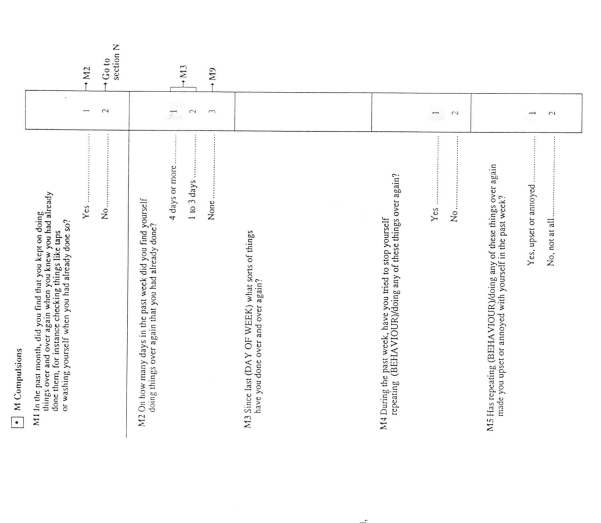

**L6 Informants who had phobic anxiety**

DNA: Others (coded 2 at K1).................. 1 →L7

**Refer to situation/thing at K3.**

Is this panic always brought on by (SITUATION/THING)?

Yes ...................... 1
No ....................... 2

L7 How long have you been having these feelings of panic as you have described?

Show card 14

less than 2 weeks................................ 1
2 weeks but less than 6 months........... 2
6 months but less than 1 year.............. 3
1 year but less than 2 years................. 4
2 years or more .................................. 5

**L8 Interviewer check:**

Sum codes which you have ringed in the shaded boxes at **L2, L3, and L4.**

Ring '0' if sum of codes is zero ... 0 →Insert score on Check card, then go to section M

or

enter score

---

**• M Compulsions**

M1 In the past month, did you find that you kept on doing things over and over again when you knew you had already done them, for instance checking things like taps or washing yourself when you had already done so?

Yes ...................... 1 →M2
No ....................... 2 →Go to section N

M2 On how many days in the past week did you find yourself doing things over again that you had already done?

4 days or more.......... 1 →M3
1 to 3 days ............... 2 →M3
None...................... 3 →M9

M3 Since last (DAY OF WEEK) what sorts of things have you done over and over again?

M14 During the past week, have you tried to stop yourself repeating (BEHAVIOUR)/doing any of these things over again?

Yes ...................... 1
No....................... 2

M5 Has repeating (BEHAVIOUR)/doing any of these things over again made you upset or annoyed with yourself in the past week?

Yes, upset or annoyed ....... 1
No, not at all .................... 2

37

38

M6 If more than one thing is repeated at M3

DNA : others .................... 1 → M7

Thinking about the past week, which of the things you mentioned did you repeat the **most** times?

Describe here → M7

M7 Since last (DAY OF WEEK), how many times did you repeat (BEHAVIOUR) when you had already done it?

| | |
|---|---|
| 3 or more repeats | 1 |
| 2 repeats | 2 |
| 1 repeat | 3 |

Refer to BEHAVIOUR at M6, if applicable

M8 How long have you been repeating (BEHAVIOUR)/any of the things you mentioned in the way which you have described?

Show card 14

| | |
|---|---|
| less than 2 weeks | 1 |
| 2 weeks but less than 6 months | 2 |
| 6 months but less than 1 year | 3 |
| 1 year but less than 2 years | 4 |
| 2 years or more | 5 |

M9 Interviewer check:

Sum codes which you have ringed in the shaded boxes at M2, M4, M5 and M7.

Ring '0' if sum of codes is zero ... 0

or

enter score → Insert score on Check card, then go to section N

---

• N Obsessions

N1 In the past month did you have any thoughts or ideas over and over again that you found unpleasant and would prefer not to think about, that still kept on coming into your mind?

| | |
|---|---|
| Yes | 1 → N2 |
| No | 2 → Go to section O |

N2 Can I check, is this the same thought or idea over and over again or are you worrying about something in general?

| | |
|---|---|
| Same thought | 1 → N3 |
| Worrying in general | 2 → See instruction below, then go to section O |

**Make a note on check flap** to go to section I to record this worry, if not already recorded.

N3 What are these unpleasant thoughts or ideas that keep coming into your mind?

**Do not probe**
**Do not press for answer**

N4 Since last (DAY OF WEEK), on how many days have you had these unpleasant thoughts?

| | |
|---|---|
| 4 days or more | 1 → N5 |
| 1 to 3 days | 2 |
| None | 3 → N9 |

N5 During the past week, have you tried to stop yourself thinking any of these thoughts?

| | |
|---|---|
| Yes | 1 |
| No | 2 |

N6 Have you become upset or annoyed with yourself when you have had these thoughts in the past week?

| | |
|---|---|
| Yes, upset or annoyed | 1 |
| Not at all | 2 |

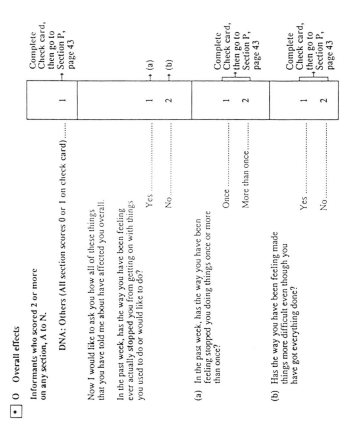

N7 In the past week, was the longest episode of having such thoughts :

Running prompt       a quarter of an hour or longer ............ 1

or was it less than this? ............ 2

N8 How long have you been having these thoughts in the way which you have just described?

Show card 14

less than 2 weeks ............ 1

2 weeks but less than 6 months ............ 2

6 months but less than 1 year ............ 3

1 year but less than 2 years ............ 4

2 years or more ............ 5

N9 Interviewer check:

Sum codes which you have ringed in the shaded boxes at N4, N5, N6 and N7.

**Ring '0' if sum of codes is zero** ...... 0

or

enter score _____

→ Insert score on Check card, then go to section O

□ O   **Overall effects**

**Informants who scored 2 or more on any section, A to N.**

DNA: Others (All section scores 0 or 1 on check card) ........ 1 → Complete Check card, then go to Section P, page 43

Now I would like to ask you how all of these things that you have told me about have affected you overall.

In the past week, has the way you have been feeling ever actually stopped you from getting on with things you used to do or would like to do?

Yes ............ 1 → (a)

No ............ 2 → (b)

(a) In the past week, has the way you have been feeling stopped you doing things once or more than once?

Once ............ 1 ⎤ Complete Check card, then go to Section P, page 43

More than once ............ 2 ⎦

(b) Has the way you have been feeling made things more difficult even though you have got everything done?

Yes ............ 1 ⎤ Complete Check card, then go to Section P, page 43

No ............ 2 ⎦

## [Page 44]

**P3.** Over the past year, have there been times when you felt that people were against you?

(a)
Yes ............ 1 →
Unsure ......... 2 →P4
No ............. 3

(a) Have there been times when you felt that people were deliberately acting to harm you or your interests?

(b)
Yes ............ 1 →
Unsure ......... 2 →P4
No ............. 3

(b) Have there been times you felt that a group of people was plotting to cause you serious harm or injury?

Yes ............ 1 → Screen Positive, Go to P6
Unsure ......... 2 →P4
No ............. 3

**P4** Over the past year, have there been times when you felt that something <u>strange</u> was going on?

(a)
Yes ............ 1 →
Unsure ......... 2 →P5
No ............. 3

(a) Did you feel it was so strange that other people would find it very hard to believe?

Yes ............ 1 → Screen Positive, Go to P6
Unsure ......... 2 →P5
No ............. 3

44

## [Page 43]

**P.** PSQ

**P1.** Over the past year, have there been times when you felt very happy indeed without a break for days on end?

(a)
Yes ............ 1 →
Unsure ......... 2 →P2
No ............. 3

(a) Was there an obvious reason for this?

Yes ............ 1 →P2
Unsure ......... 2
No ............. 3
(b)

(b) Did your relatives or friends think it was strange or complain about it?

Yes ............ 1 → Screen Positive, Go to P6
Unsure ......... 2 →P2
No ............. 3

**P2.** Over the past year, have you ever felt that your thoughts were directly interfered with or controlled by some outside force or person?

(a)
Yes ............ 1 →
Unsure ......... 2 →P3
No ............. 3

(a) Did this come about in a way that many people would find hard to believe, for instance, through telepathy?

Yes ............ 1 → Screen Positive, Go to P6
Unsure ......... 2 →P3
No ............. 3

43

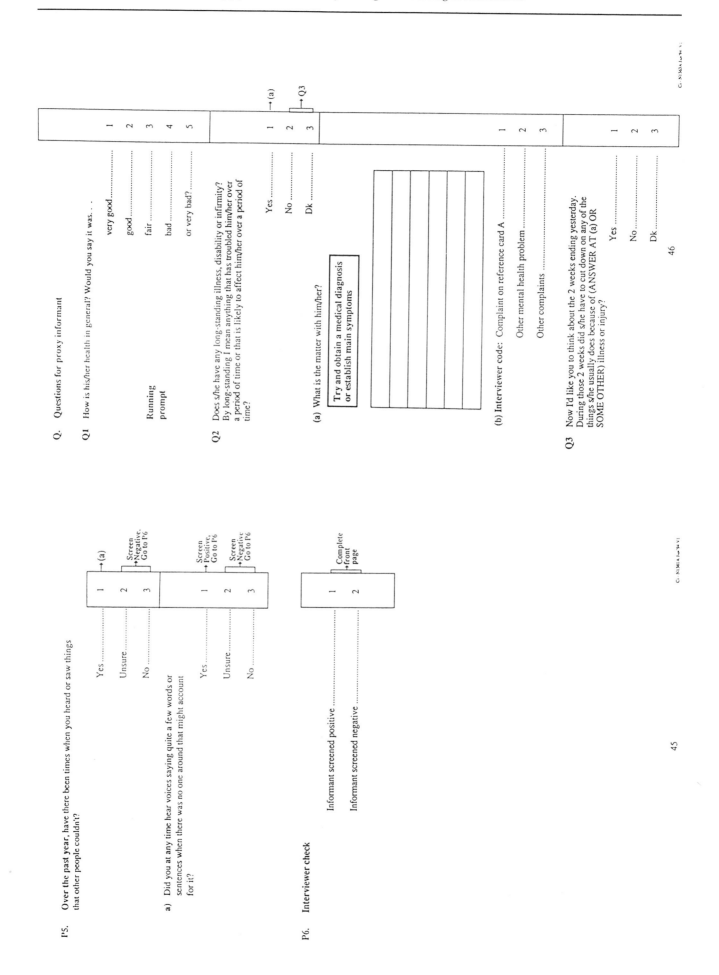

**Q. Questions for proxy informant**

Q1 How is his/her health in general? Would you say it was. . .

Running prompt

| | |
|---|---|
| very good | 1 |
| good | 2 |
| fair | 3 |
| bad | 4 |
| or very bad? | 5 |

Q2 Does s/he have any long-standing illness, disability or infirmity? By long-standing I mean anything that has troubled him/her over a period of time or that is likely to affect him/her over a period of time?

| | | |
|---|---|---|
| Yes | 1 | → (a) |
| No | 2 | |
| Dk | 3 | Q3 |

(a) What is the matter with him/her?

> Try and obtain a medical diagnosis or establish main symptoms

(b) Interviewer code:

| | |
|---|---|
| Complaint on reference card A | 1 |
| Other mental health problem | 2 |
| Other complaints | 3 |

Q3 Now I'd like you to think about the 2 weeks ending yesterday. During those 2 weeks did s/he have to cut down on any of the things s/he usually does because of (ANSWER AT (a) OR SOME OTHER) illness or injury?

| | |
|---|---|
| Yes | 1 |
| No | 2 |
| Dk | 3 |

46

P5. **Over the past year, have there been times when you heard or saw things that other people couldn't?**

| | | |
|---|---|---|
| Yes | 1 | → (a) |
| Unsure | 2 | |
| No | 3 | Screen Negative, Go to P6 |

a) Did you at any time hear voices saying quite a few words or sentences when there was no one around that might account for it?

| | | |
|---|---|---|
| Yes | 1 | Screen Positive, Go to P6 |
| Unsure | 2 | |
| No | 3 | Screen Negative, Go to P6 |

P6. **Interviewer check**

| | | |
|---|---|---|
| Informant screened positive | 1 | Complete front page |
| Informant screened negative | 2 | |

45

62

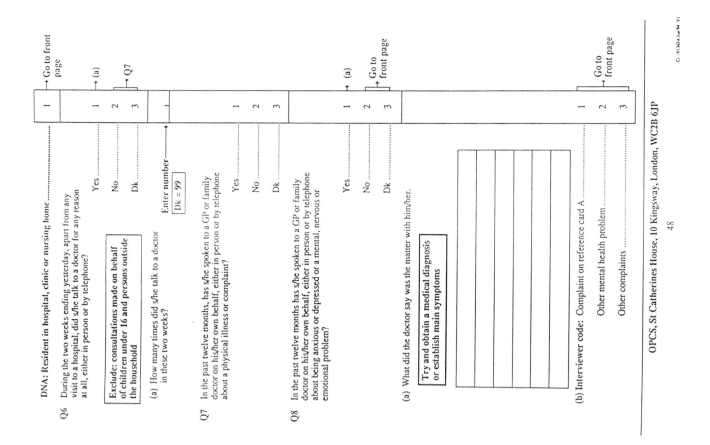

DNA: Resident in hospital, clinic or nursing home ..... 1 → Go to front page

Q6  During the two weeks ending yesterday, apart from any visit to a hospital, did s/he talk to a doctor for any reason at all, either in person or by telephone?

Yes ..... 1 → (a)
No ..... 2
Dk ..... 3 → Q7

Exclude: consultations made on behalf of children under 16 and persons outside the household

(a) How many times did s/he talk to a doctor in these two weeks?

Enter number ..... 
Dk = 99

Q7  In the past twelve months, has s/he spoken to a GP or family doctor on his/her own behalf, either in person or by telephone about a physical illness or complaint?

Yes ..... 1
No ..... 2
Dk ..... 3

Q8  In the past twelve months has s/he spoken to a GP or family doctor on his/her own behalf, either in person or by telephone about being anxious or depressed or a mental, nervous or emotional problem?

Yes ..... 1 → (a)
No ..... 2 → Go to front page
Dk ..... 3

(a) What did the doctor say was the matter with him/her.

Try and obtain a medical diagnosis or establish main symptoms

(b) Interviewer code:  Complaint on reference card A ..... 1
Other mental health problem ..... 2
Other complaints ..... 3 → Go to front page

OPCS, St Catherines House, 10 Kingsway, London, WC2B 6JP

48

G. N136A/...94 V1

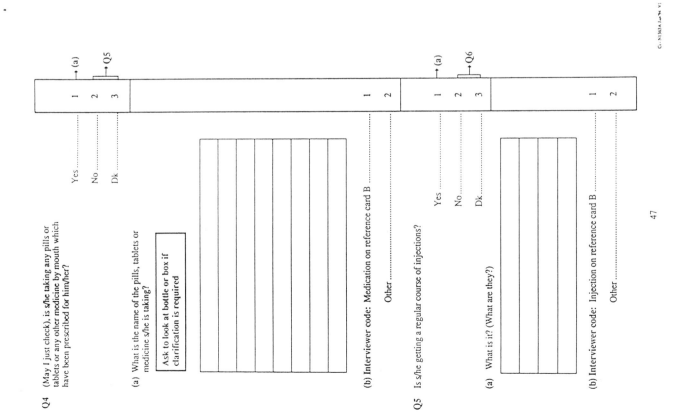

Q4  (May I just check), is s/he taking any pills or tablets or any other medicine by mouth which have been prescribed for him/her?

Yes ..... 1 → (a)
No ..... 2
Dk ..... 3 → Q5

(a) What is the name of the pills, tablets or medicine s/he is taking?

Ask to look at bottle or box if clarification is required

(b) Interviewer code:  Medication on reference card B ..... 1
Other ..... 2

Q5  Is s/he getting a regular course of injections?

Yes ..... 1 → (a)
No ..... 2 → Q6
Dk ..... 3

(a) What is it? (What are they?)

(b) Interviewer code:  Injection on reference card B ..... 1
Other ..... 2

47

G. N136A/...94 V1

F

N1363

Person

Stick serial number label

**Check card**   Enter Scores :

A   Somatic symptoms

B   Fatigue

C   Concentration and forgetfulness

D   Sleep problems

E   Irritability

F   Worry about physical health

G   Depression

H   Depressive ideas

I   Worry

J   Anxiety

K   Phobias

L   Panic

M   Compulsions

N   Obsessions

Total score: sections A to N
→ Enter here

Go to section P,
page 43.

Note: Threshold
is 12 or more

O. N1363 Part 4 V1

## Reference Card A

- Auditory hallucinations
- Bipolar affective disorder
- Catatonic schizophrenia
- Chronic schizophrenia
- Hallucinations
- Hearing voices
- Hebephrenic schizophrenia
- Hypomania
- Mania
- Manic depression
- Manic depressive psychosis
- Mental illness
- Mentally disturbed
- Mild psychosis
- Mild schizophrenia
- Mood swings
- Neuroleptic
- Paranoia
- Paranoid schizophrenia
- Psychosis
- Psychotic related disorder
- Psychotic tendencies
- Schizo-affective disorder
- Schizophrenia
- Schizophrenic affective disorder
- Simple schizophrenia
- Voices

G. NISAK May 94 VI

## Reference card B

| | | |
|---|---|---|
| Anquil | Haldol decanoate | Priadel |
| Benperidol | Halperidol | Prochlorperazine |
| Camcolit | Largactil | Promazine hydrochloride |
| Chlorpromazine | Liskonum | Redeptin |
| Clopixol acuphase | Litarex | Remoxipride |
| Clopixol | Lithium | Roxiam |
| Clozapine | Loxapac | Serenace |
| Clozaril | Loxapine | Sparine |
| Depixol | Melleril | Stelazine |
| Dolmatil | Methotrimeprazine | Sulphiride |
| Dozic | Modecate | Sulpitil |
| Droleptan | Moditen | Thioridazine |
| Droperidol | Moditen ethanate | Trifluoperazine |
| Fentazin | Neulactil | Trifluperidol |
| Fluanxol | Nozinan | Zuclopenthixol dihydrochloride |
| Flupenthixol | Orap | Zuclopenthixol acetate |
| Flupenthixol decanoate | Oxypertine | Zuclopenthixol decanoate |
| Fluphenazine hydrochloride | Pericyazine | |
| Fluphenazine decanoate | Perphenazine | *Antipsychotic drugs* |
| Fluphenazine enanthate | Phasal | *Antipsychotic injections* |
| Fluspirilene | Pimozide | *Depot injections* |
| Fortunan | Piportil | *Antimanic drugs* |
| Haldol | Pipothiazine palmitate | |

G. NISAK May 94 VI

N1363  Yellow Schedule  B

IN CONFIDENCE

| Stick serial number label | | Person | | Date of Interview | 9 | 4 |

○1

- - - - - - - - - - - - - - - - - - - - -

**Complete at end of interview.**

(i) Type of interview:

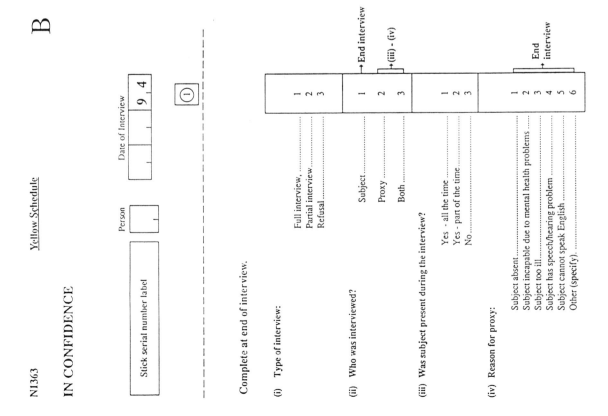

|  |  |
|---|---|
| Full interview, | 1 → **End interview** |
| Partial interview | 2 |
| Refusal | 3 |

(ii) Who was interviewed?

|  |  |
|---|---|
| Subject | 1 |
| Proxy | 2 → (iii) - (iv) |
| Both | 3 |

(iii) Was subject present during the interview?

|  |  |
|---|---|
| Yes - all the time | 1 |
| Yes - part of the time | 2 |
| No | 3 |

(iv) Reason for proxy:

|  |  |
|---|---|
| Subject absent | 1 |
| Subject incapable due to mental health problems | 2 |
| Subject too ill | 3 → **End interview** |
| Subject has speech/hearing problem | 4 |
| Subject cannot speak English | 5 |
| Other (specify) | 6 |

O-13658 Jun 94  V2

1

66

## A  Long-standing illness

**A1**  Informant has long-standing illness or saw a GP about a mental, nervous or emotional problem

DNA:Informants coded 2 at qn.11, page 6 **and** qn.17, page 8, Schedule A
Proxy informants coded 2 or 3 at Q2, page 46 **and** Q8, page 48, Schedule A ...............

[ ] **1** → Go to Section B page **4**

Refer to complaints in Schedule A:
For informants, see qn.11a, page 6 **and** qn.17a, page 8;
For proxy informants, see Q2a, page 46 **and** Q8a, page 48.

Earlier you told me about (COMPLAINT(s)).
I'd now like to ask you a few more questions about this.

Transcribe details of complaint(s) from Schedule A.

| COMPLAINT No. → | 1 | 2 | 3 | 4 | 5 | 6 | 7 | 8 |
|---|---|---|---|---|---|---|---|---|
| (a) Name of complaint or Describe main symptoms [Try and obtain medical diagnosis] | | | | | | | | |
| | OFF USE | OFF USE | OFF USE | OFF USE | OFF USE | OFF USE | OFF USE | OFF USE |
| (b) How old were you when your (COMPLAINT) started? Enter AGE — Code 00 if from birth Code 99 if DK | □□ | □□ | □□ | □□ | □□ | □□ | □□ | □□ |
| (c) For how long has your (COMPLAINT) been at its present level? Enter no. of years OR if less than 1 year Enter no. of months (less than 1 month = 00) | □□ □□ | □□ □□ | □□ □□ | □□ □□ | □□ □□ | □□ □□ | □□ □□ | □□ □□ |
| (d) In the past week, did your (COMPLAINT) actually stop you from getting on with the things you usually do or would like to do? [*]  Yes...... / No...... | 1 / 2 | 1 / 2 | 1 / 2 | 1 / 2 | 1 / 2 | 1 / 2 | 1 / 2 | 1 / 2 |

O.1636/10-'94 V2

2

3

## B. Medication and treatment

**B1** DNA: No oral medication or injections (coded 2 at qns.13 and 14, page 7 or if proxy, coded 2 or 3 at Q4 and Q5, page 47, Schedule A).............. [1] → B2

Ring column number when appropriate →

Columns: 1, 2, 3, 4, 5, 6, 7, 8

(a) Transcribe list of pills, medication or injections from questions 13(a) and 14(a), page 7, or Q4(a) and Q5(a), page 47, Schedule A

> Try and establish brand name. If necessary, ask informant to look at name on bottle or box

*(Each column:* Injection: Ring → [1]  OFF USE)

(b) What is its/their strength?

> If strength of pills not known, describe colour and note what is written on tablet

*(Each column:* OFF USE)

(c) How many/much are you supposed to have each day?

Enter number of pills/mls/injections per day →

OR if less than 1 one a day

Enter number of pills/mls/injections per month →
(Less than one per month = 00)

Spontaneous: Take as needed.................. [1]

(d) For what condition do you take them?

> Obtain medical diagnosis AND describe main symptoms

*(Each column:* OFF USE)

(e) How long have you been having this medication?

Enter number of years →

OR if less than 1 year

Enter number of months →
(Less than 1 month = 0 0)

O.1618 I wk 94 V2

| Ring column number when appropriate→ | 1 | 2 | 3 | 4 | 5 | 6 | 7 | 8 |
|---|---|---|---|---|---|---|---|---|
| **(f)** Do you sometimes not take your medication even though you should?  Yes........  No........ | 1 → (g)  2 → (i) | 1 → (g)  2 → (i) | 1 → (g)  2 → (i) | 1 → (g)  2 → (i) | 1 → (g)  2 → (i) | 1 → (g)  2 → (i) | 1 → (g)  2 → (i) | 1 → (g)  2 → (i) |
| **(g)** When was the last time this happened?  *Prompt as necessary*  Less than 1 week ago  At least 1 week but less than 1 month ago  At least 1 month ago | 1  2  3 | 1  2  3 | 1  2  3 | 1  2  3 | 1  2  3 | 1  2  3 | 1  2  3 | 1  2  3 |
| **✳ (h)** What was the reason for this?  *Code all that apply*  Forgot  Didn't need it  Don't like to take drugs  Side effects  Other | 1  2  3  4  5 | 1  2  3  4  5 | 1  2  3  4  5 | 1  2  3  4  5 | 1  2  3  4  5 | 1  2  3  4  5 | 1  2  3  4  5 | 1  2  3  4  5 |
| **(i)** Do you sometimes take more medication/pills than the stated dose?  Yes........  No........ | 1 → (j)  2 → (l) | 1 → (j)  2 → (l) | 1 → (j)  2 → (l) | 1 → (j)  2 → (l) | 1 → (j)  2 → (l) | 1 → (j)  2 → (l) | 1 → (j)  2 → (l) | 1 → (j)  2 → (l) |
| **(j)** When was the last time this happened?  *Prompt as necessary*  Less than 1 week ago  At least 1 week but less than 1 month ago  At least 1 month ago | 1  2  3 | 1  2  3 | 1  2  3 | 1  2  3 | 1  2  3 | 1  2  3 | 1  2  3 | 1  2  3 |
| **✳ (k)** What was the reason for this?  *Code all that apply*  Needed more to control symptoms  Deliberate overdose  Other | 1  2  3 | 1  2  3 | 1  2  3 | 1  2  3 | 1  2  3 | 1  2  3 | 1  2  3 | 1  2  3 |

6

7

O.116916613 V2

**Columns 4–8 (page 9)**

| Question | 4 | 5 | 6 | 7 | 8 |
|---|---|---|---|---|---|
| **(m)** DNA: already asked about this condition in a previous column | 1 → col 5 or B2 | 1 → col 6 or B2 | 1 → col 7 or B2 | 1 → col 8 or B2 | 1 → B2 |
| Have you had any other medication or treatment for (CONDITION AT (l)) which you don't have now  Yes | 1 → (n) | 1 → (n) | 1 → (n) | 1 → (n) | 1 → (n) |
| No | 2 → (p) | 2 → (p) | 2 → (p) | 2 → (p) | 2 → (p) |
| **(n)** Did you stop this treatment on your own accord or on professional advice?  Own accord | 1 → (o) | 1 → (o) | 1 → (o) | 1 → (o) | 1 → (o) |
| Professional advice | 2 → (p) | 2 → (p) | 2 → (p) | 2 → (p) | 2 → (p) |
| **(o)** What made you decide to stop this treatment?  Code all that apply  Did not work/were not strong enough | 1 | 1 | 1 | 1 | 1 |
| Side effects | 2 | 2 | 2 | 2 | 2 |
| Other | 3 | 3 | 3 | 3 | 3 |
| **(p)** Have you ever been offered any other medication or treatment for (CONDITION) which you refused?  Yes | 1 → (q) | 1 → (q) | 1 → (q) | 1 → (q) | 1 → (q) |
| No | 2 → col 5 or B2 | 2 → col 6 or B2 | 2 → col 7 or B2 | 2 → col 8 or B2 | 2 → B2 |
| **(q)** What was it? |  |  |  |  |  |
|  | OFF USE | OFF USE | OFF USE | OFF USE | OFF USE |
| **(r)** Why did you refuse it?  Code all that apply  Worry about side effects | 1 | 1 | 1 | 1 | 1 |
| Don't like medication/treatment | 2 | 2 | 2 | 2 | 2 |
| Other | 3 | 3 | 3 | 3 | 3 |

**Columns 1–3 (page 8)**

| Question | 1 | 2 | 3 |
|---|---|---|---|
| Ring column number when appropriate → |  |  |  |
| (l) Transcribe condition from each column in the order recorded at (d), pages 4 and 5 |  |  |  |
| **(m)** DNA: already asked about this condition in a previous column | X | 1 → col 3 or B2 | 1 → col 4 or B2 |
| Have you had any other medication or treatment for (CONDITION AT (l)) which you don't have now  Yes |  | 1 → (n) | 1 → (n) |
| No |  | 2 → (p) | 2 → (p) |
| **(n)** Did you stop this treatment on your own accord or on professional advice?  Own accord | 1 → (o) | 1 → (o) | 1 → (o) |
| Professional advice | 2 → (p) | 2 → (p) | 2 → (p) |
| **(o)** What made you decide to stop this treatment?  Code all that apply  Did not work/were not strong enough | 1 | 1 | 1 |
| Side effects | 2 | 2 | 2 |
| Other | 3 | 3 | 3 |
| **(p)** Have you ever been offered any other medication or treatment for (CONDITION) which you refused?  Yes | 1 → (q) | 1 → (q) | 1 → (q) |
| No | 2 → col 2 or B2 | 2 → col 3 or B2 | 2 → col 4 or B2 |
| **(q)** What was it? |  |  |  |
|  | OFF USE | OFF USE | OFF USE |
| **(r)** Why did you refuse it?  Code all that apply  Worry about side effects | 1 | 1 | 1 |
| Don't like medication/treatment | 2 | 2 | 2 |
| Other | 3 | 3 | 3 |

9

8

## B2 (page 10)

**B2** (*) At the moment are you having any counselling or therapy?

Yes...... 1 →(a)
No...... 2 →Section C page 12

Ring column no. when appropriate →

| | 1 | 2 | 3 |
|---|---|---|---|
| (a) What type of counselling or therapy are you having at the moment? | OFF USE | OFF USE | OFF USE |
| (b) How often do you have this counselling/therapy? | | | |
| Enter no. of treatments per month → | | | |
| OR if less than one per month | | | |
| Enter no. of treatments per year → | | | |
| Spontaneous: when needed........... | 1 | 1 | 1 |
| (c) How long have you been having this counselling/therapy? | | | |
| Enter number of years → | | | |
| OR if less than 1 year | | | |
| Enter number of months → (less than 1 month = 0 0) | | | |
| (d) For what condition are you having this counselling/therapy? | | | |
| Obtain medical diagnosis AND describe main symptoms | | | |
| (e) Interviewer check: Is condition at B2(d) mentioned at B1(d), pages 4 and 5? | OFF USE | OFF USE | OFF USE |
| Yes ......... | 1 → col 2 or C1 | 1 → col 3 or C1 | 1 → C1 |
| No......... | 2 → (f) | 2 → (f) | 2 → (f) |

## (page 11)

Ring column number when appropriate →

| | 1 | 2 | 3 |
|---|---|---|---|
| (f) DNA: Already asked about this condition in a previous column...... | X | 1 → col 3 or C1 | 1 → C1 |
| Have you had any other treatment or medication for (CONDITION AT d) which you don't have now? Yes......... | 1 → (g) | 1 → (g) | 1 → (g) |
| No........ | 2 → (i) | 2 → (i) | 2 → (i) |
| (g) Did you stop this treatment on your own accord or on professional advice? On own accord.. | 1 → (h) | 1 → (h) | 1 → (h) |
| Professional advice.. | 2 → (i) | 2 → (i) | 2 → (i) |
| (*) (h) What made you decide to stop this treatment? Code all that apply — Did not work/was not strong enough...... | 1 | 1 | 1 |
| Side effects........ | 2 | 2 | 2 |
| Other....... | 3 | 3 | 3 |
| (i) Have you ever been offered any other treatment or medication for (CONDITION AT d) which you refused? Yes......... | 1 → (j) | 1 → (j) | 1 → (j) |
| No......... | 2 → col 2 or C1 | 2 → col 3 or C1 | 2 → C1 |
| (j) What was it? | | | |
| (*) (k) Why did you refuse it? Code all that apply — Worry about side effects........ | OFF USE / 1 | OFF USE / 1 | OFF USE / 1 |
| Don't like medication/treatment...... | 2 | 2 | 2 |
| Other........ | 3 | 3 | 3 |

10

11

**C1A** To those in hospital, clinic or nursing home

DNA: Others ................ 1 → C2

Which of the people listed on this card have you seen in this (ESTABLISHMENT) in the past 12 months/since you have been here?

Show card 15

For each person seen, ask (a)

(a) How often do you see (PERSON)?

Show card 17

| | Yes | No | (a) How often do you see (PERSON) | | | | |
| --- | --- | --- | --- | --- | --- | --- | --- |
| | | | 4+ times a week | 2-3 times a week | Once a week | At least once a month | Less than once a month |
| Psychiatrist/Psychotherapist........ | 1 | 2 | 1 | 2 | 3 | 4 | 5 |
| Other consultant/hospital doctor .......... | 1 | 2 | 1 | 2 | 3 | 4 | 5 |
| Psychiatric Nurse............... | 1 | 2 | 1 | 2 | 3 | 4 | 5 |
| Social worker/Counsellor....... | 1 | 2 | 1 | 2 | 3 | 4 | 5 |
| Occupational Therapist (OT) ...... | 1 | 2 | 1 | 2 | 3 | 4 | 5 |
| Psychologist............... | 1 | 2 | 1 | 2 | 3 | 4 | 5 |
| Voluntary worker............ | 1 | 2 | 1 | 2 | 3 | 4 | 5 |
| Don't know................. | 9 | | | | | | |

---

**C Health, social and voluntary care services**

**GP consultations** DNA: In hospital, clinic or nursing home ...... 1 → C1A page 13

**C1** During the two weeks ending yesterday, apart from any visit to a hospital, did you talk to a GP or family doctor on your own behalf, either in person or by telephone?

Yes ................ 1 → (a)

No ................ 2 → C2, page 14

(a) How many times have you talked to your GP or family doctor in the past two weeks?

Enter number of times ............ → (b)

Ask (b) to (d) for the last 4 consultations (1 = most recent)

| | 1 | 2 | 3 | 4 |
| --- | --- | --- | --- | --- |
| Ring consultation number —— | | | | |
| (b) When you spoke to the doctor (on...occasion) did you talk about: | | | | |
| a physical illness or complaint.. | 1 | 1 | 1 | 1 |
| or about being anxious or depressed, or a mental, nervous or emotional problem?............ | 2 | 2 | 2 | 2 |
| Spontaneous: Both of these............. | 3 | 3 | 3 | 3 |
| (c) Were you satisfied or dissatisfied with the consultation? | | | | |
| Satisfied............ | 1→col 2 or C2 | 1→col 3 or C2 | 1→col 4 or C2 | 1→C2 |
| Dissatisfied............ | 2 → (d) | 2 → (d) | 2 → (d) | 2 → (d) |
| (d) In what way were you dissatisfied? | | | | |
| Doctor does not listen, not interested, ignores me............ | 1 | 1 | 1 | 1 |
| Informant thinks treatment was inappropriate............. | 2 | 2 | 2 | 2 |
| Informant not given tests, treatment or hospitalisation... | 3 | 3 | 3 | 3 |
| Doctor said there was nothing wrong or nothing s/he could do.... | 4 | 4 | 4 | 4 |
| Other............. | 5 | 5 | 5 | 5 |

Running prompt

Code all that apply

**Ring in-patient episode number** →

| (c) Who referred you to (the other) hospital? | 1 | 2 | 3 | 4 |
|---|---|---|---|---|
| GP | 01 | 01 | 01 | 01 |
| Community Psychiatric Nurse | 02 | 02 | 02 | 02 |
| Social worker | 03 | 03 | 03 | 03 |
| Psychiatrist | 04 | 04 | 04 | 04 |
| Via casualty (A and E) | 05 | 05 | 05 | 05 |
| Via law courts/Probation Service or Police | 06 | 06 | 06 | 06 |
| Self-admitted | 07 | 07 | 07 | 07 |
| Other | 08 | 08 | 08 | 08 |

(d) When you were there which people did you see?

[Show card 15] [Exclude nurse with non specific duties]

| Code all that apply | 1 | 2 | 3 | 4 |
|---|---|---|---|---|
| Psychiatrist/Psychotherapist | 01 | 01 | 01 | 01 |
| Other consultant or hospital doctor | 02 | 02 | 02 | 02 |
| Psychiatric Nurse | 03 | 03 | 03 | 03 |
| Social Worker/Counsellor | 04 | 04 | 04 | 04 |
| Occupational Therapist (OT) | 05 | 05 | 05 | 05 |
| Psychologist | 06 | 06 | 06 | 06 |
| Voluntary worker | 07 | 07 | 07 | 07 |

15

In patient stays (in other hospitals)

C2 During the past year, that is since (DATE) have you been in (another) hospital or anywhere else as an in-patient, overnight or longer for treatment or tests?

[Include sight or hearing problems]

[Exclude giving birth]

Yes ...... 1 → C3
No ........ 2 → C5, page 16

C3 In the past 12 months, how many separate stays have you had in (another) hospital or anywhere else as an in-patient?

Enter number of stays →

C4 Ask (a) to (d) for the last 4 in-patient episodes (1=most recent)

Ring in-patient episode number →

(a) How many nights altogether were you there on the (.....) stay?

Enter number of nights →

(b) Were you there because of

Running prompt
- a physical health problem
- or a mental nervous or emotional problem?

Spontaneous: Both

| | 1 | 2 | 3 | 4 |
|---|---|---|---|---|
| | 1→col 2 or C5 | 1→col 3 or C5 | 1→col 4 or C5 | 1→C5 |
| | 2 ](c) | 2 ](c) | 2 ](c) | 2 ](c) |
| | 3 | 3 | 3 | 3 |

14

73

Ring column no. when appropriate ⟶

C6(d) Which of these people did you normally see at this hospital/clinic? [Exclude nurse with non specific duties]

Show card 15

| | 1 | 2 | 3 | 4 |
|---|---|---|---|---|
| Psychiatrist/Psychotherapist | 01 | 01 | 01 | 01 |
| Other consultant/hospital doctor | 02 | 02 | 02 | 02 |
| Code all that apply — Psychiatric Nurse | 03 | 03 | 03 | 03 |
| Social worker/Counsellor | 04 | 04 | 04 | 04 |
| Occupational Therapist (OT) | 05 | 05 | 05 | 05 |
| Psychologist | 06 | 06 | 06 | 06 |
| Other | 07 | 07 | 07 | 07 |
| (e) Are you currently attending (PLACE)? — Yes | 1→col 2 or C7; 2→(f) | 1→col 3 or C7; 2→(f) | 1→col 4 or C7; 2→(f) | 1→C7; 2→(f) |
| No | | | | |
| (f) Have you stopped going of your own accord or were you discharged? — On own accord | 1 | 1 | 1 | 1 |
| Discharged | 2 | 2 | 2 | 2 |

17

---

Out-patient episodes

C5 (Apart from seeing your own doctor/when you stayed in hospital) In the past 12 months have you been to a hospital or clinic or anywhere else for treatment or check-ups?

[Include visits to hospitals, day hospitals, clinics and private consulting rooms]

[Include attendance at day centres for treatment. Exclude attendance at day centres for leisure. Exclude sheltered workshops]

Yes ⟶ 1 →(a)
No ⟶ 2 → C7, page 18

(a) How many different places have you been for out-patient or day patient visits in the past year?

Enter number of places ⟶ [ ]

C6 For each place attended, ring column number and ask (a) to (f)

Ring column no. ⟶

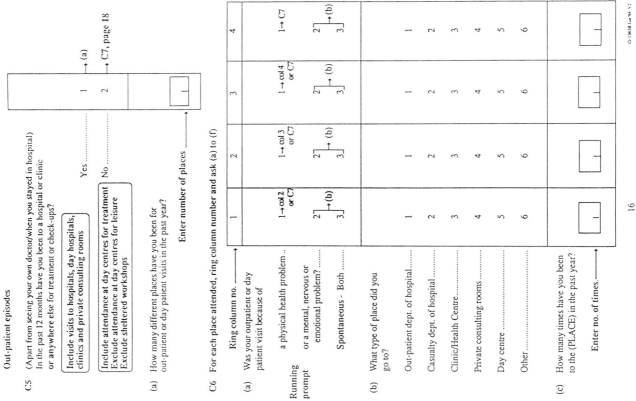

| | 1 | 2 | 3 | 4 |
|---|---|---|---|---|
| (a) Was your outpatient or day patient visit because of — a physical health problem | 1→col 2 or C7 | 1→col 3 or C7 | 1→col 4 or C7 | 1→C7 |
| Running prompt — or a mental, nervous or emotional problem? | 2 →(b) | 2 →(b) | 2 →(b) | 2 →(b) |
| Spontaneous - Both | 3 | 3 | 3 | 3 |
| (b) What type of place did you go to? — Out-patient dept. of hospital | 1 | 1 | 1 | 1 |
| Casualty dept. of hospital | 2 | 2 | 2 | 2 |
| Clinic/Health Centre | 3 | 3 | 3 | 3 |
| Private consulting rooms | 4 | 4 | 4 | 4 |
| Day centre | 5 | 5 | 5 | 5 |
| Other | 6 | 6 | 6 | 6 |
| (c) How many times have you been to the (PLACE) in the past year? — Enter no. of times | [ ] | [ ] | [ ] | [ ] |

16

DNA: In hospital, clinic or nursing home ...........

C7 Here is a list of people who visit people in their homes to give them help and support when they need it.
Have any of these people visited you in the past year?

Yes ........... 1 → (a)
No ........... 2 → C8, page 20

Show card 16

Ring person no. Code all that apply →

| | Community Psychiatric Nurse | Occupational Therapist | Social Worker | Psychiatrist | Home care worker/ Home help | Voluntary Worker | Second Voluntary Worker |
|---|---|---|---|---|---|---|---|
| | 1 | 2 | 3 | 4 | 5 | 6 | 7 |

(a) How often does (PERSON) come?

Show card 17

| | CPN | OT | SW | Psych | Home help | Vol | 2nd Vol |
|---|---|---|---|---|---|---|---|
| 4 or more times a week | 1 | 1 | 1 | 1 | 1 | 1 | 1 |
| 2 or 3 times a week | 2 | 2 | 2 | 2 | 2 | 2 | 2 |
| Once a week | 3 | 3 | 3 | 3 | 3 | 3 | 3 |
| Less often than once a week but at least once a month | 4 | 4 | 4 | 4 | 4 | 4 | 4 |
| Less often than once a month | 5 | 5 | 5 | 5 | 5 | 5 | 5 |

(b) How satisfied or dissatisfied are you with the help or support (PERSON) gives you?

\* Are you

| | CPN | OT | SW | Psych | Home help | Vol | 2nd Vol |
|---|---|---|---|---|---|---|---|
| very satisfied | 1 | 1 | 1 | 1 | 1 | 1 | 1 |
| Running prompt — fairly satisfied | 2 | 2 | 2 | 2 | 2 | 2 | 2 |
| fairly dissatisfied | 3 | 3 | 3 | 3 | 3 | 3 | 3 |
| or very dissatisfied? | 4 | 4 | 4 | 4 | 4 | 4 | 4 |

(c) Ask for voluntary worker(s) if applicable

Which voluntary organisation does (PERSON) come from?

| | CPN | OT | SW | Psych | Home help | Voluntary Worker | Second Voluntary Worker |
|---|---|---|---|---|---|---|---|
| Voluntary worker does not come from any organisation | | | | | | 1 | 1 |
| MIND | | | | | | 2 | 2 |
| Manic Depression Fellowship | | | | | | 3 | 3 |
| Phobic Action/Society | | | | | | 4 | 4 |
| National Schizophrenia Fellowship | | | | | | 5 | 5 |
| Cruse | | | | | | 6 | 6 |
| Alcohol concern | | | | | | 7 | 7 |
| Standing conference on Drug Abuse | | | | | | 8 | 8 |
| Other | | | | | | 9 | 9 |

**C8** [Show card 18]

In the past year, have you been offered any help or support from any of the people listed on this card, or indeed any other service, **which you turned down?**

| | |
|---|---|
| Yes | 1 → (a) |
| No | 2 → C9 |

(a) What sort of help/service were you offered?

Code all that apply

| | |
|---|---|
| Community Psychiatric Nurse | 1 |
| Occupational Therapist/Industrial Therapist | 2 |
| Social Worker/Counselling Service | 3 |
| Psychiatrist | 4 |
| Home care worker/Home help | 5 |
| Voluntary Worker | 6 |
| Other | 7 |

* (b) Did you turn it down because you did not want or need the help or for some other reason?

Code all that apply

| | |
|---|---|
| Did not want/need help | 1 |
| Could not face it/handle it | 2 |
| Did not like people/not the right people offering help | 3 |
| Didn't think it could/would help | 4 |
| Inconvenient time or location | 5 |
| Other reason | 6 |

20

---

DNA: **In hospital, clinic or nursing home** ... 1 → D8, page 24

**C9** Sometimes people do not see a doctor or other professional about mental, nervous or emotional problems when perhaps they should. In the past year did you decide not to see a doctor or other professional when either you or people around you thought you should?

| | |
|---|---|
| Yes | 1 → (a) |
| No | 2 → Section D |

* (a) Thinking about the last time this happened, what were your reasons for not going to a doctor or other professional?

Write verbatim and then code

Code all that apply

| | |
|---|---|
| Didn't know who to go to or where to go | 01 |
| Did not think anyone could help | 02 |
| Hour inconvenient/didn't have the time | 03 |
| Thought problem would get better by itself | 04 |
| Too embarrassed to discuss it with anyone | 05 |
| Afraid what family/friends would think | 06 |
| Family or friends objected | 07 |
| Afraid of consequences (treatment, tests, hospitalisation, sectioned) | 08 |
| Afraid of side effects of any treatment | 09 |
| Didn't think it was necessary/No problem | 10 |
| A problem one should be able to cope with | 11 |
| Other | 12 |

→ Section D

21

## D. Practical activities

[*]

**Do you have any difficulty . . . .**

| | | (a) Do you have any difficulty | | | (a) Do you need anyone to help you ( . . . . . ) | | (b) Who helps you . . . Code all that apply from list |
|---|---|---|---|---|---|---|---|
| | | Yes | No | DNA | Yes | No | |
| D1 | With personal care such as dressing, bathing, washing, or using the toilet? — with personal care? | 1 | 2 | 3 | 1 | 2 | ☐ ☐ ☐ |
| D2 | Getting out and about or using transport? — getting out and about? | 1 | 2 | 3 | 1 | 2 | ☐ ☐ ☐ |
| D3 | With medical care such as taking medicines or pills, having injections or changes of dressing? — with medical care? | 1 | 2 | 3 | 1 | 2 | ☐ ☐ ☐ |
| D4 | With household activities like preparing meals, shopping, laundry and housework? — with household activities? | 1 | 2 | 3 | 1 | 2 | ☐ ☐ ☐ |
| D5 | With practical activities such as gardening, decorating, or doing household repairs? — with practical activities? | 1 | 2 | 3 | 1 | 2 | ☐ ☐ ☐ |
| D6 | Dealing with paperwork, such as writing letters, sending cards or filling in forms? — dealing with paperwork? | 1 | 2 | 3 | 1 | 2 | ☐ ☐ ☐ |
| D7 | Managing money, such as budgeting for food or paying bills? — managing money? | 1 | 2 | 3 | 1 | 2 | ☐ ☐ ☐ |

| Code | |
|---|---|
| 00 | No one |
| 01 | Spouse/cohabitee |
| 02 | Brother/sister (incl. in-law) |
| 03 | Son/daughter (incl. in-law) |
| 04 | Parent (incl. in-law) |
| 05 | Grandparent (incl. in-law) |
| 06 | Grandchild (incl. in-law) |
| 07 | Other relative |
| 08 | Boyfriend/girlfriend |
| 09 | Friend |
| 10 | CPN/Nurse |
| 11 | Occupational Therapist |
| 12 | Social worker |
| 13 | Home care worker/home help |
| 14 | Voluntary worker |
| 15 | Landlord/landlady |
| 16 | Paid domestic help |
| 17 | Paid nurse |
| 18 | Bank manager |
| 19 | Solicitor |
| 20 | Other person (specify) |

22

23

## Recent Life Events

DNA: Proxy interviews.......... | 1 | → Go to Section E, page 28

The following questions are about events or problems which may have happened to you during the past 6 months which might have caused you distress and to seek help

> Use card 19 if subject not alone, otherwise, ask D8 to D13
>
> Then ask (a) to (g) if coded 1 at main

### Columns (a)–(c)

| | Yes / No | (a) When did this happen? More than 6 months = 6, Less than 1 month = 0. No of months since event | (b) Was there anyone, among your family or friends, who understood what this felt like? | (c) And were you able to talk about it openly and get support and understanding? |
|---|---|---|---|---|
| **D8** In the past 6 months, have you yourself suffered from a serious illness, injury or an assault? | 1  2 | [ ] | Yes 1 → (c) / No 2 → (d) | Yes 1 / No 2 |
| **D9** (In the past 6 months,) has a serious illness, injury or an assault happened to a close relative? | 1  2 | [ ] | Yes 1 → (c) / No 2 → (d) | Yes 1 / No 2 |
| **D10** (In the past 6 months,) has a parent, spouse (or partner), child, brother or sister of yours died? | 1  2 | [ ] | Yes 1 → (c) / No 2 → (d) | Yes 1 / No 2 |
| **D11** (In the past 6 months,) has a close family friend or another relative died, such as an aunt, cousin or grandparent? | 1  2 | [ ] | Yes 1 → (c) / No 2 → (d) | Yes 1 / No 2 |
| **D12** (In the past 6 months,) have you had a separation due to marital difficulties or broken off a steady relationship? | 1  2 | [ ] | Yes 1 → (c) / No 2 → (d) | Yes 1 / No 2 |
| **D13** (In the past 6 months,) have you had a serious problem with a close friend, neighbour or relative? | 1  2 | [ ] | Yes 1 → (c) / No 2 → (d) | Yes 1 / No 2 |

24

### Columns (d)–(g)

| | (d) Did you get any professional help, for this, that is from someone other than family or friends? | (e) Did you try to get help for this, from any professional? | (f) Was this because you didn't know where to get the help you wanted from or because you felt you didn't need any professional help? | (g) Was it help with practical things or did you need someone to talk things over with? |
|---|---|---|---|---|
| | Yes 1 → (g) / No 2 → (e) | Yes 1 → (g) / No 2 → (f) | DK where 1 → (g) / Didn't need help 2 → See D9 | Practical 1  Talk over 2  Both 3 → See D9 |
| | Yes 1 → (g) / No 2 → (e) | Yes 1 → (g) / No 2 → (f) | DK where 1 → (g) / Didn't need help 2 → See D10 | Practical 1  Talk over 2  Both 3 → See D10 |
| | Yes 1 → (g) / No 2 → (e) | Yes 1 → (g) / No 2 → (f) | DK where 1 → (g) / Didn't need help 2 → See D11 | Practical 1  Talk over 2  Both 3 → See D11 |
| | Yes 1 → (g) / No 2 → (e) | Yes 1 → (g) / No 2 → (f) | DK where 1 → (g) / Didn't need help 2 → See D12 | Practical 1  Talk over 2  Both 3 → See D12 |
| | Yes 1 → (g) / No 2 → (e) | Yes 1 → (g) / No 2 → (f) | DK where 1 → (g) / Didn't need help 2 → See D13 | Practical 1  Talk over 2  Both 3 → See D13 |
| | Yes 1 → (g) / No 2 → (e) | Yes 1 → (g) / No 2 → (f) | DK where 1 → (g) / Didn't need help 2 → Go to D14 | Practical 1  Talk over 2  Both 3 → Go to D14 |

25

Now I'd like to ask you about some other events or problems which may have happened to you during the past 6 months.

> **If subject is in hospital, home or clinic start at D16, or use show card 20b.**

> **Use card 20a if subject not alone, otherwise, ask D14 to D18**
> **Then ask (a) to (g) if coded 1 at main**

| | Yes / No | (a) When did this happen? More than 6 months = 6 Less than 1 month = 0 — No of months since event | (b) Was there anyone, among your family or friends, who understood what this felt like? Yes / No | (c) And were you able to talk about it openly and get support and understanding? Yes / No |
|---|---|---|---|---|
| **D14** In the past 6 months, were you made redundant or sacked from your job? | 1   2 | ☐ | 1 →(c)   2 →(d) | 1   2 |
| **D15** (In the past 6 months,) were you seeking work without success for more than one month? | 1   2 | ☐ | 1 →(c)   2 →(d) | 1   2 |
| **D16** (In the past 6 months,) did you have a major financial crisis, such as losing the equivalent of 3 months income? | 1   2 | ☐ | 1 →(c)   2 →(d) | 1   2 |
| **D17** (In the past 6 months,) did you have problems with the police involving a court appearance? | 1   2 | ☐ | 1 →(c)   2 →(d) | 1   2 |
| **D18** (In the past 6 months,) was something you valued lost or stolen? | 1   2 | ☐ | 1 →(c)   2 →(d) | 1   2 |

26

| (d) Did you get any professional help for this, that is from someone other than family or friends? Yes / No | (c) Did you try to get help for this, from any professional? Yes / No | (f) Was this because you didn't know where to get the help you wanted from or because you felt you didn't need any professional help? DK where / Didn't need help | (g) Was it help with practical things or did you need for someone to talk things over with? Practical / Talk over / Both |
|---|---|---|---|
| 1 →(g)   2 →(c) | 1 →(g)   2 →(f) | 1 →(g)   2 → See D15 | 1   2   3 → See D15 |
| 1 →(g)   2 →(e) | 1 →(g)   2 →(f) | 1 →(g)   2 → See D16 | 1   2   3 → See D16 |
| 1 →(g)   2 →(e) | 1 →(g)   2 →(f) | 1 →(g)   2 → See D17 | 1   2   3 → See D17 |
| 1 →(g)   2 →(e) | 1 →(g)   2 →(f) | 1 →(g)   2 → See D18 | 1   2   3 → See D18 |
| 1 →(g)   2 →(e) | 1 →(g)   2 →(f) | 1 →(g)   2 → Go to Section E | 1   2   3 → Go to Section E |

27

## E  Social Life

**E1.** The next few questions are about how you spend your leisure time.

When you are here, what sorts of things do you usually do during your leisure time?

Show card 21

Code all that apply

| | | (a) Do on | |
|---|---|---|---|
| | | Share | own |
| Entertaining friends or relatives | 01 | ╳ | |
| Writing letters/telephoning | 02 | ╳ | |
| Reading books and newspapers | 03 | ╳ | |
| TV/radio | 04 | 1 | 2 |
| Listening to music | 05 | 1 | 2 |
| Hobbies inc. art and crafts, knitting, playing a musical instrument, writing poetry | 06 | 1 | 2 |
| Gardening | 07 | 1 | 2 |
| DIY/ car maintenance | 08 | 1 | 2 |
| Games inc. cards, computer games, betting and gambling | 09 | 1 | 2 |
| Other indoor leisure pursuits | 10 | 1 | 2 |
| Spontaneous: No leisure time/no indoor leisure pursuits | 99 | → Go to E3 | |

(a) Ask for each activity informant does **except** for 'entertaining friends or relatives', 'writing letters/telephoning' and 'reading books and newspapers':

Refer to activity and ask:

Is this an interest which you share with someone else and usually do together or do you usually do it on your own?

Ring code in column (a) above.
Then go to E2.

---

**E2.** What sorts of things do you usually do during your leisure time away from here?

Show card 22

Code all that apply

| | | (a) Do on | |
|---|---|---|---|
| | | Share | own |
| Visiting friends or relatives | 01 | ╳ | |
| Pubs, restaurants | 02 | 1 | 2 |
| Night clubs, discos | 03 | 1 | 2 |
| Clubs, organisations | 04 | 1 | 2 |
| Classes, lectures | 05 | 1 | 2 |
| Going for a walk, walking the dog | 06 | 1 | 2 |
| Sports inc. keep fit, cycling, swimming, football and horse riding | 07 | 1 | 2 |
| Sports as a spectator | 08 | 1 | 2 |
| Cinema, theatre, concerts | 09 | 1 | 2 |
| Bingo, amusement arcades | 10 | 1 | 2 |
| Bookmakers, betting and gambling | 11 | 1 | 2 |
| Shopping | 12 | 1 | 2 |
| Church | 13 | 1 | 2 |
| Political activities | 14 | 1 | 2 |
| Library | 15 | 1 | 2 |
| Other outdoor leisure pursuits | 16 | 1 | 2 |
| Spontaneous: Does not go out or not allowed out | 98 | | |
| Spontaneous: No leisure time/no outdoor leisure pursuits | 99 | → Go to E3 | |

(a) Ask for each activity informant does **except** for 'visiting friends or relatives':

Refer to activity and ask:

Is this an interest which you share with someone else and usually do/go to together or do you usually do it/go on your own?

Ring code in column (a) above.

**E3.** Do you go to any of these places for <u>social</u> activities?

| | | Yes | No |
|---|---|---|---|
| Individual prompt | (a) Day centre? | 1 | 2 |
| | (b) Club for people with physical health problems? | 1 | 2 |
| | (c) Club for people with mental health problems? | 1 | 2 |
| | (d) Any other types of social club? | 1 | 2 |

**E4.** Do you regularly go to ......

| | Yes | No |
|---|---|---|
| (a) an Adult Education Centre? | 1 | 2 |
| (b) an Adult Training Centre? | 1 | 2 |

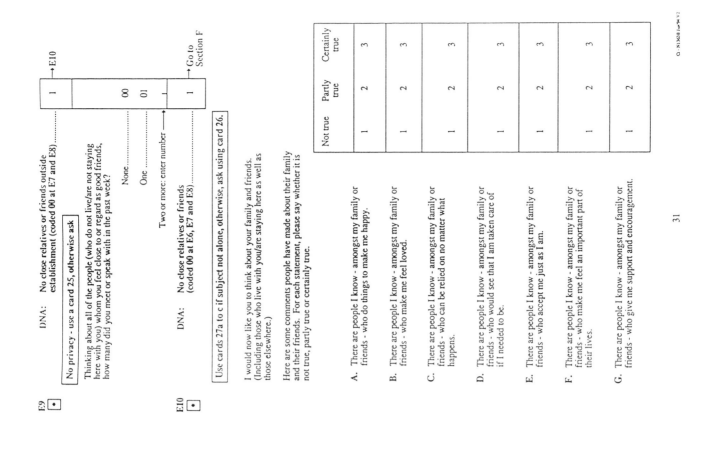

**E9.** [*]

DNA: No close relatives or friends outside establishment (coded **00** at **E7** and **E8**) ........ 1 → E10

No privacy - use a card 25, otherwise ask

Thinking about all of the people (who do not live/are not staying here with you) whom you feel close to or regard as good friends, how many did you meet or speak with in the past week?

None ........ 00

One ........ 01

Two or more: enter number ___ ↑

**E10.** [*]

DNA: No close relatives or friends (coded **00** at **E6, E7** and **E8**) ........ 1 → Go to Section F

Use cards 27a to c if subject not alone, otherwise, ask using card 26.

I would now like you to think about your family and friends. (Including those who live with you/are staying here as well as those elsewhere.)

Here are some comments people have made about their family and their friends. For each statement, please say whether it is not true, partly true or certainly true.

| | Not true | Partly true | Certainly true |
|---|---|---|---|
| A. There are people I know - amongst my family or friends - who do things to make me happy. | 1 | 2 | 3 |
| B. There are people I know - amongst my family or friends - who make me feel loved. | 1 | 2 | 3 |
| C. There are people I know - amongst my family or friends - who can be relied on no matter what happens. | 1 | 2 | 3 |
| D. There are people I know - amongst my family or friends - who would see that I am taken care of if I needed to be. | 1 | 2 | 3 |
| E. There are people I know - amongst my family or friends - who accept me just as I am. | 1 | 2 | 3 |
| F. There are people I know - amongst my family or friends - who make me feel an important part of their lives. | 1 | 2 | 3 |
| G. There are people I know - amongst my family or friends - who give me support and encouragement. | 1 | 2 | 3 |

31

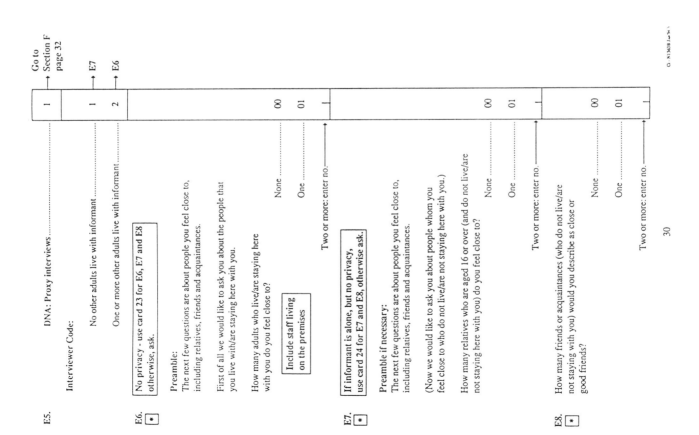

**E5.** DNA: Proxy interviews ........ 1 → Go to Section F page 32

Interviewer Code:

No other adults live with informant ........ 1 → E7

One or more other adults live with informant ........ 2 → E6

**E6.** [*]

No privacy - use card 23 for E6, E7 and E8 otherwise, ask.

Preamble:
The next few questions are about people you feel close to, including relatives, friends and acquaintances.

First of all we would like to ask you about the people that you live with/are staying here with you.

How many adults who live/are staying here with you do you feel close to?

Include staff living on the premises

None ........ 00

One ........ 01

Two or more: enter no. ___ ↑

**E7.** [*]

If informant is alone, but no privacy, use card 24 for E7 and E8, otherwise ask.

Preamble if necessary:
The next few questions are about people you feel close to, including relatives, friends and acquaintances.

(Now we would like to ask you about people whom you feel close to who do not live/are not staying here with you.)

How many relatives who are aged 16 or over (and do not live/are not staying here with you) do you feel close to?

None ........ 00

One ........ 01

Two or more: enter no. ___ ↑

**E8.** [*]

How many friends or acquaintances (who do not live/are not staying with you) would you describe as close or good friends?

None ........ 00

One ........ 01

Two or more: enter no. ___ ↑

30

## F    Education and Employment Status

**F1.** At what age did you finish your continuous full-time education at school or college?

| | |
|---|---|
| Not yet finished | 1 |
| Never went to school | 2 |
| 14 or under | 3 |
| 15 | 4 |
| 16 | 5 |
| 17 | 6 |
| 18 | 7 |
| 19 or over | 8 |

**F2.** Please look at this card and tell me whether you have passed any of the qualifications listed. **Look down the list and tell me the first one you come to that you have passed.**

Show card 28

Code first that applies

| | |
|---|---|
| Degree (or degree level qualification) | 1 |
| Teaching qualification <br> HNC/HND, BEC/TEC Higher, BTEC Higher <br> City and Guilds Full Technological Certificate | 2 |
| Nursing qualifications (SRN, SCM, RGN, RM <br> RHV, Midwife | 3 |
| 'A' levels/SCE higher <br> ONC/OND/BEC/TEC **not** higher <br> City and Guilds Advanced/Final level | 3 |
| 'O' level passes (Grade A - C if after 1975) <br> GCSE (Grades A - C) <br> CSE Grade 1 <br> SCE Ordinary (Bands A - C) <br> Standard Grade (Level 1 - 3) <br> SLC Lower <br> SUPE Lower or Ordinary <br> School Certificate or Matric. <br> City and Guilds Craft/Ordinary level | 4 |
| CSE Grades 2 - 5 <br> GCE 'O' level (Grades D & E if after 1975) <br> GCSE (Grades D, E, F, G) <br> SCE Ordinary (Bands D & E) <br> Standard Grade (Level 4,5) <br> Clerical or commercial qualifications <br> Apprenticeship | 5 |
| CSE ungraded | 6 |
| Other qualifications (specify) | 7 |
| No qualifications | 8 |

**F5. Interviewer check**

| | | |
|---|---|---|
| Had a job last week (coded 01 at F3 or 02 at F3(a)) | 1 | → F8 |
| Unemployed waiting to take up a job (coded 03 at F3(a)(i)) | 2 | → F6 |
| Unemployed looking for work (coded 04 or 05 at F3(a)(i)) | 3 | → F7 |
| Others - economically inactive (coded 06 to 10 at F3(a)(i)) | 4 | |

**F6. Unemployed waiting to take up a job**

Apart from the job you are waiting to take up, have you ever had a paid job or done any paid work?

| | | |
|---|---|---|
| Yes | 1 | → F8 |
| No | 2 | |

**F7. All others unemployed and economically inactive**

(May I check) have you ever had a paid job or done any paid work?

| | | |
|---|---|---|
| Yes | 1 | → F8 |
| No | 2 | → See F20, page **41** |

35

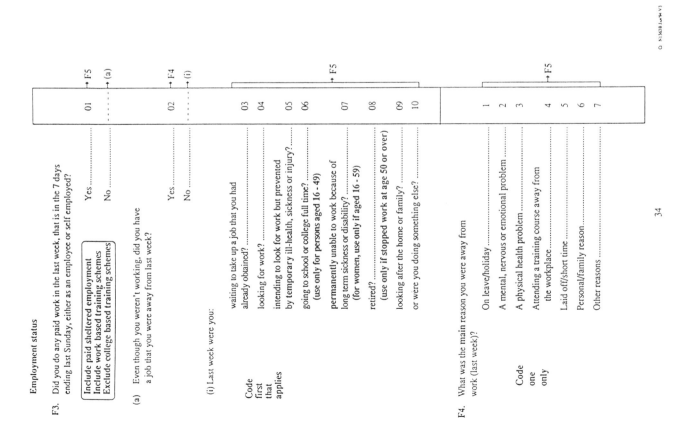

**Employment status**

**F3.** Did you do any paid work in the last week, that is in the 7 days ending last Sunday, either as an employee or self employed?

> Include paid sheltered employment
> Include work based training schemes
> Exclude college based training schemes

| | | |
|---|---|---|
| Yes | 01 | → F5 |
| No | | → (a) |

(a) Even though you weren't working, did you have a job that you were away from last week?

| | | |
|---|---|---|
| Yes | 02 | → F4 |
| No | | → (i) |

(i) Last week were you:

Code first that applies

| | |
|---|---|
| waiting to take up a job that you had already obtained? | 03 |
| looking for work? | 04 |
| intending to look for work but prevented by temporary ill-health, sickness or injury? | 05 |
| going to school or college full time? (use only for persons aged 16 - 49) | 06 |
| permanently unable to work because of long term sickness or disability? (for women, use only if aged 16 - 59) | 07 |
| retired? (use only if stopped work at age 50 or over) | 08 |
| looking after the home or family? | 09 |
| or were you doing something else? | 10 |

(→ F5)

**F4.** What was the main reason you were away from work (last week)?

Code one only

| | |
|---|---|
| On leave/holiday | 1 |
| A mental, nervous or emotional problem | 2 |
| A physical health problem | 3 |
| Attending a training course away from the workplace | 4 |
| Laid off/short time | 5 |
| Personal/family reason | 6 |
| Other reasons | 7 |

(→ F5)

34

F11. To those with a job last week (coded 1 at F5, page 35)

DNA: Unemployed/Economically Inactive ...... 1 → See F18, page 40

A. For employees (main job/government scheme)
How long have you been with your present employer (up to yesterday)?

B. For self-employed (main job)
How long have you been self-employed (up to yesterday)?

Show Card 29 and prompt as necessary

| | |
|---|---|
| Less than 4 weeks ...... | 01 |
| 4 weeks but less than 3 months ...... | 02 |
| 3 months but less than 6 months ...... | 03 |
| 6 months but less than 12 months ...... | 04 |
| 12 months but less than 2 years ...... | 05 |
| 2 years but less than 3 years ...... | 06 |
| 3 years but less than 5 years ...... | 07 |
| 5 years but less than 10 years ...... | 08 |
| 10 years but less than 15 years ...... | 09 |
| 15 years but less than 20 years ...... | 10 |
| 20 years but less than 25 years ...... | 11 |
| 25 years but less than 30 years ...... | 12 |
| 30 years but less than 35 years ...... | 13 |
| 35 years but less than 40 years ...... | 14 |
| 40 years or more ...... | 15 |

F12. A. For employees (main job/government scheme)
(Introduce if on short time/lay-off:
I'd like to ask about your hours when you are not on short time/laid off...)

How many hours a week do you usually work (in your main job/government scheme), that is excluding meal breaks and overtime?

Check with informant that this is excluding any paid or unpaid overtime

NO OF HOURS excluding meal breaks and overtime

B. For self-employed, (main job)
(Introduce if on short time/lay-off:
I'd like to ask about your hours when you are not on short time/laid off ...)

How many hours a week in total do you usually work (in your main job), that is excluding meal breaks but including any overtime

Check with informant that this is total hours including any paid or unpaid overtime

TOTAL HOURS excluding meal breaks

If work pattern not based on a week, give average over a few months

37

F8. If employed
(i) What was your job last week?

If not employed
(ii) What was your most recent job?

(iii) What is the job you are waiting to take up?

If retired
(iv) What was your main job?

Job title:

Description:

Industry:

SOC
IND

(a) Informant's Definition
Full-time ...... 1
Part-time ...... 2

(b) Employee ...... 1 → F9
Self-employed ...... 2 → F10

F9 (a) If employee ask or record
Manager ...... 1
Foreman/supervisor ...... 2
other employee ...... 3

(b) How many employees work(ed) in the establishment
1 - 24 ...... 1
25 - 499 ...... 2
500 or more ...... 3

(c) Do/did you work in sheltered employment such as with:
Running Prompt
Remploy ...... 1
a local authority ...... 2
a blind association ...... 3
a voluntary association ...... 4
or in a sheltered place with an ordinary employer? ...... 5
DK/None of these ...... 6

F10 If self employed
Do/did you employ other people?
Yes, PROBE: 1 - 24 ...... 1
25 - 499 ...... 2
500 or more ...... 3
No employees ...... 4

36

**F13.**

DNA: Proxy interview ........... 1 → See F26, page 43

Earlier I was asking you about how you had been feeling in the past month.

Has your health or the way you have been feeling caused you to take time off work in the past year?

Yes .......... 1 → (a)
No ........... 2 → F14

(a) How many days in the past year have you taken off work?

Enter number of days →

[Weekends falling within a period of sickness must be included]

38

**F14.** **To those with a job last week but temporarily not working because of a mental or physical health problem (coded 2 or 3 at F4, page 34)**

DNA: Others ........... 1 → Section G, page 45

How long have you been off work?

Less than 2 weeks .......... 1
2 weeks, less than 1 month .......... 2
1 month, less than 3 months .......... 3
3 months, less than 6 months .......... 4
6 months or more .......... 5

**F15. If employee**

DNA: Self-employed (coded 2 at F8(b), page 36) ........... 4 → F16

* Do you expect to return to your present employer?

Yes .......... 1 → (a)
No .......... 2
Not sure .......... 3 → F16

(a) Do you expect to return to the same job?

Yes .......... 1 → Section G, page 45
No .......... 2
DK .......... 3

**F16.** Do you expect to be fit to work again?

Yes .......... 1 → F17
No .......... 2
Not sure .......... 3 → Section G, page 45

**F17.** Will you look for another paid job in the future?

Yes .......... 1 → Section G, page 45
No .......... 2
DK .......... 3 → (a)

(a) Why will/may you not look for another job?

Code all that apply

No suitable jobs: general employment situation .......... 1
No suitable jobs: due to health problems .......... 2
Too old .......... 3
Other .......... 4 → Section G, page 45

39

**F18. If not working but has worked**

  DNA: Never worked (coded 2 at F6, page 35) ...... 1 → See F20

  How old were you when you left your last paid job?

  Enter age _____ 1 → Section G, page 45

**F19.**

  * DNA: Proxy interview..... 1 → See F20

  Did a mental, nervous or emotional problem have anything to do with your leaving your last job?

  Yes ................. 1 → (a)
  No .................. 2 → See F20

  (a) DNA: Self-employed in last job (coded 2 at F8 (b) page 36) ...... 1 → See F20

  Did your employer ask you to leave or did you leave of your own accord?

  Employer asked ............. 1 ┐
  Left of own accord ......... 2 ┘ → See F20

**F20.**  DNA: Proxy interview ................................ 1 → Section G, page 45

  DNA: Retired (code 08 at F3(a)(i), page 34) ............. 1 → Section G, page 45

  **If not working but not retired**

  * Is the reason that you are not working at present that ...

  Code first that applies

  the way you have been feeling makes it impossible for you to do any kind of paid work? ........................ 1 → (a)
  a physical health problem makes it impossible for you to do any kind of paid work? ........................ 2 → F21
  you have not found a suitable paid job? ........................ 3 → F21
  or because you do not want or need a paid job? ........................ 4 → Section G, page 45
  Other ........................ 5 → F21

  * (a) May I just check, would you be able to do some kind of sheltered or part-time work if it were available, or is this impossible?

  Priority code

  Could do part-time work ......... 1 ┐
  Could do sheltered work ......... 2 ┘ → F21
  Impossible to do work ........... 3 → Section G, page 45

**F21.** (May I just check) Are you looking for a job at the moment?

  * Yes ........................ 1 → F23
    No ......................... 2 → (a)

  * (a) Have you looked for a job at all (since you last worked)?

    Yes ....................... 1 → F22
    No ........................ 2 → (i)

  * (i) Why have you not looked for a job?

  Code all that apply

  No suitable jobs around - general employment situation ................ 1 → Section G, page 45
  No suitable jobs for someone with subject's health problem ............ 2
  Other .................................. 3

**F22.** Why have you stopped looking for jobs?

  * Code all that apply

  No suitable jobs around - general employment situation ................ 1
  No suitable jobs for someone with subject's health problem ............ 2
  Other .................................. 3

40

41

Blank page

F23. (Since you last worked) have you (ever) done any of the following to help get a job:

| | Yes | No |
|---|---|---|
| Visited a local Job Centre? | 1 | 2 |
| Talked to a Careers Officer? | 1 | 2 |
| Talked to a Disablement Resettlement Officer (DRO)? | 1 | 2 |

**Individual Prompt**

F24. Do you think that the way you have been feeling over the past month makes it more difficult for you than for other people to find a job?

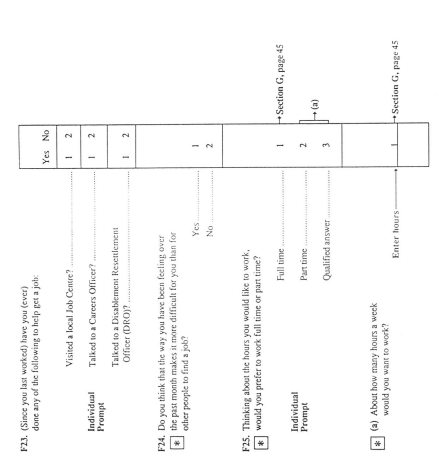

Yes ............... 1 → Section G, page 45

No ............... 2

F25. Thinking about the hours you would like to work, would you prefer to work full time or part time?

Full time ............... 1 → Section G, page 45

Part time ............... 2 → (a)

Qualified answer ............... 3

**Individual Prompt**

(a) About how many hours a week would you want to work?

Enter hours ⟶ | 1 | → Section G, page 45

**G** Finances

**G.0.** Do you look after and control your own financial affairs, perhaps with some help, or does someone else have control of them?

| | |
|---|---|
| Controls own financial affairs | 1 → See G1 |
| Someone else has financial control/ Only receives "pocket money" | 2 → (a) |

**Partial control is coded 2**

(a) Who is in control of your financial affairs?

**Code all that apply**

| | |
|---|---|
| Court of protection | 01 |
| Power of (enduring) attornery | 02 |
| Appointeeship (e.g. relative, friend or solicitor) or Finance officer at establishment | 03 |
| Informant's bank | 04 |
| DSS Direct payments | 05 |
| Other (including informal arrangements) (Specify) | 06 → Go to Section H page 49 |
| Don't know | 99 |

Blank page

45

44

88

DNA: In hospital, clinic or nursing home ...... 1 → Section II page 49

**G1.** Are you receiving any of the state benefits shown on this card?

Yes ...... 1 → Code (a) - (f)

No ...... 2 → G2

| Show card 30 |
|---|

|  | Yes | No |
|---|---|---|
| (a) Child benefit? | 1 | 2 → ask (i) |
| (i) As well as child benefit, do you receive the one-parent benefit? | 1 | 2 |
| (b) Family credit? | 1 | 2 |
| (c) N.I. Retirement pension or Old Age pension? | 1 | 2 |
| (d) Income Support? | 1 | 2 |
| (e) N.I. Sickness benefit (Not Employer's Statutory sick pay) | 1 | 2 |
| (f) Unemployment benefit? | 1 | 2 |

46

**G2.** (In addition) are you receiving any of the State benefits listed on this card or any other N.I. or State benefit (for example, war benefits or maternity allowance)?

Yes ...... 1 → Code (a) - (m)

No ...... 2 → G3

| Show card 31 |
|---|

|  | Yes | No |
|---|---|---|
| (a) Widow's pension or War Widow's pension? | 1 | 2 |
| (b) Any other State Widow's benefit (eg Widowed Mother's allowance)? [Exclude Widow's benefit] | 1 | 2 |
| (c) War disablement pension? | 1 | 2 |
| (d) Invalidity pension, Invalidity benefit or allowance? | 1 | 2 |
| (e) Severe disablement allowance? | 1 | 2 |
| (f) Mobility allowance? | 1 | 2 |
| (g) Industrial disablement allowance? | 1 | 2 |
| (h) Attendance allowance? | 1 | 2 |
| (i) Disability Living allowance? | 1 | 2 |
| (j) Disability Working allowance? | 1 | 2 |
| (k) Invalid care allowance? | 1 | 2 |
| (l) Maternity allowance? | 1 | 2 |
| (m) Anything else? (Specify) | 1 | 2 |

47

## Other Income

**G3.** (In addition to these), do you receive income from any of the sources on this card?

Show card 32

Yes ......... 1 → Code (a) - (f)
No ......... 2 → G4

| | Yes | No |
|---|---|---|
| (a) Earned Income/salary? | 1 | 2 |
| (b) Income from self-employment? | 1 | 2 |
| (c) Pension from a former employer? | 1 | 2 |
| (d) Interest from savings, building society, investment dividends from shares etc? | 1 | 2 |
| (e) Other kinds of regular allowances from outside the household (eg alimony, annuity, educational grant)? | 1 | 2 |
| (f) Any other source?(specify) | 1 | 2 |

**G4.** Could you please look at this card and tell me which group represents your own personal gross income from all sources mentioned?

By gross income, I mean income from all sources before deductions for income tax and National Insurance.

Show card 33

Enter group number
or
DK ......... 98
Refused ......... 99 → See section H page 49

---

## II Smoking

**II1** Have you ever smoked a cigarette, a cigar, or a pipe?

DNA: Proxy interview ......... 1 → Complete front page
Yes ......... 1 → II2
No ......... 2 → Go to Section I, page 52

**II2.** Do you smoke cigarettes at all nowadays?

Yes ......... 1 → H3
No ......... 2 → H10

**H3.** About how many cigarettes a day do you usually smoke at weekends?

Less than 1
No. smoked a day ......... 00

**H4.** And about how many cigarettes a day do you usually smoke on weekdays?

Less than 1
No. smoked a day ......... 00

**H5.** Do you mainly smoke

**Running prompt**
**Code one only**

filter-tipped cigarettes ......... 1 → H6
or plain or untipped cigarettes ......... 2 → H6
or hand-rolled cigarettes? ......... 3 → H7

**H6.** Which brand of cigarette do you usually smoke?

Enter details

Full brand name

Size e.g, King, luxury, regular

Filter tipped or plain

INTERVIEWER: Code from reference card C

Not on list ......... 1 → H7

**H7.** How easy or difficult would you find it to go without smoking for a whole day?

Running prompt

| | |
|---|---|
| Very easy | 1 |
| Fairly easy | 2 |
| Fairly difficult | 3 |
| Very difficult? | 4 |
| DK | 5 |

**H8.** Would you like to give up smoking altogether?

| | |
|---|---|
| Yes | 1 |
| No | 2 |
| DK | 3 |

**H9.** How soon after waking do you usually smoke your first cigarette of the day?

| | | |
|---|---|---|
| Less than 5 minutes | 1 | |
| 5 - 14 minutes | 2 | |
| 15 - 29 minutes | 3 | |
| 30 minutes but less than 1 hour | 4 | |
| 1 hour but less than 2 hours | 5 | |
| 2 hours or more | 6 | → H11 |

50

**H10.** Have you ever smoked cigarettes regularly?

| | | |
|---|---|---|
| Yes | 1 | → (a) |
| No | 2 | → H12 |

**(a)** About how many cigarettes did you smoke in a day when you smoked them regularly?

| | |
|---|---|
| Less than 1 | 00 |
| No. smoked a day | |

**(b)** How long ago did you stop smoking cigarettes regularly?

| | | |
|---|---|---|
| Less than 6 months ago | 1 | |
| 6 months but less than a year ago | 2 | |
| 1 year but less than 2 years ago | 3 | |
| 2 years but less than 5 years ago | 4 | |
| 5 years but less than 10 years ago | 5 | |
| 10 years or more ago | 6 | → H11 |

**H11.** How old were you when you started to smoke cigarettes regularly?

Enter age

| | | |
|---|---|---|
| Spontaneous: Never smoked cigarettes regularly | 00 | → H12 |

**H12.** Do you smoke at least one cigar of any kind per month nowadays?

| | | |
|---|---|---|
| Yes | 1 | → (a) |
| No | 2 | → (b) |

**(a)** About how many cigars do you usually smoke in a week?

| | | |
|---|---|---|
| Less than 1 | 00 | → See H13 |
| No. smoked a week | | |

**(b)** Have you ever regularly smoked at least one cigar of any kind per month?

| | | |
|---|---|---|
| Yes | 1 | → See H13 |
| No | 2 | |

**H13.** To all men who have ever smoked (Coded 1 at H1)

| | | |
|---|---|---|
| DNA: Women | 1 | Go to Section I page 52 |

Do you smoke a pipe at all nowadays?

| | | |
|---|---|---|
| Yes | 1 | → H14 |
| No | 2 | Go to Section I page 52 |

**H14.** Have you ever smoked a pipe regularly?

| | | |
|---|---|---|
| Yes | 1 | Go to Section I page 52 |
| No | 2 | |

51

# I  Drinking

**I1.** I'm now going to ask you a few questions about what you drink - that is, if you do drink.

Do you ever drink alcohol nowadays, including drinks you brew or make at home?

| | | |
|---|---|---|
| Yes | 1 | →I5 |
| No | 2 | →I2 |

**I2.** Could I just check, does that mean you never have an alcoholic drink nowadays, or do you have an alcoholic drink very occasionally, perhaps for medicinal purposes or on special occasions like Christmas or New Year?

| | | |
|---|---|---|
| Very occasionally | 1 | →I5 |
| Never | 2 | →I3 |

**I3.** Have you always been a non-drinker, or did you stop drinking for some reason?

| | | |
|---|---|---|
| Always a non-drinker | 1 | →I4(a) |
| Used to drink but stopped | 2 | →I4(b) |

**I4(a). Always a non drinker**

[*] Why is that?

Code all that apply

| | | |
|---|---|---|
| Religious reasons | 1 | |
| Don't like it | 2 | |
| Parent's advice | 3 | Go to self completion, page 2, then complete front page |
| Health reasons | 4 | |
| Can't afford it | 5 | |
| Other | 6 | |

**I4(b). Used to drink but stopped**

[*] What would you say was the main reason you stopped drinking?

Code all that apply

| | | |
|---|---|---|
| Religious reasons | 1 | |
| Don't like it | 2 | |
| Parent's advice | 3 | Go to self completion, page 2, then complete front page |
| Health reasons | 4 | |
| Can't afford it | 5 | |
| Other | 6 | |

**I5.** I'm going to read out a few descriptions about the amounts of alcohol people drink, and I'd like you to say which one fits you best.
Would you say you:

[*]

**Running prompt**

| | | |
|---|---|---|
| hardly drink at all | 1 | |
| drink a little | 2 | |
| drink a moderate amount | 3 | |
| drink quite a lot | 4 | |
| or drink heavily? | 5 | |
| DK | 6 | |

→I6

**17.** Ask for each group of alcoholic drinks coded 1 - 7 at I6 (drunk in the last 12 months)

How much . . . . . . . . have you usually drunk on any one day?

→ Enter the amount

Leave blank for the groups of drink that the informant has not drunk at all in the last 12 months.

EXCLUDE: Any non-alcoholic drinks
Any low-alcohol drinks
(other than shandy)

| | Amount drunk on any one day during the last 12 months |
|---|---|
| Shandy (exluding bottles/cans) | half pints |
| Beer, lager, stout, cider | half pints OR / large cans, OR / small cans |
| Spirits or liqueurs (e.g. gin, whisky, rum, brandy, vodka, advocaat) | singles (Count doubles as 2 singles) |
| Sherry or martini (including port, vermouth, cinzano, dubonnet) | glasses |
| Wine (inc. babycham, champagne) | glasses |
| Any other alcoholic drinks? | |

If the informant had any other type of alcoholic drink at I6, record the name of the drink again and enter the amount usually drunk on any one day.

Specify name of drink
. . . . . . . . . . . . . . . . . . . . . . . . . . . . .

OFF. USE

Go to 18

55

O: N136/8 1oc'94 V2

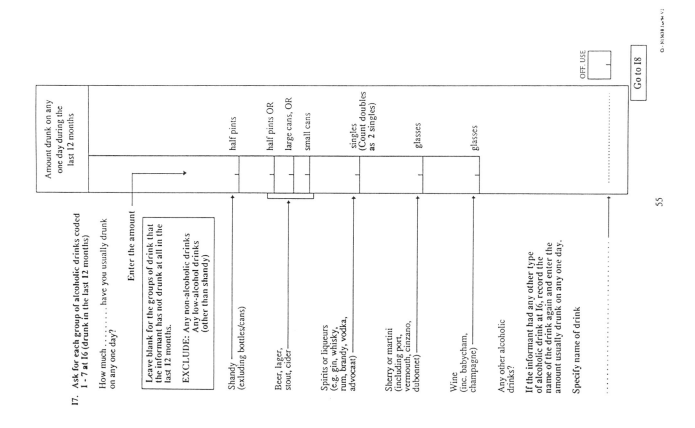

---

**16.** Show Card 34 and ask for each group of alcoholic drinks listed below:

How often have you had a drink of . . . . . . during the last 12 months?

Ring the appropriate number

EXCLUDE: Any non-alcoholic drinks.
Any low-alcohol drinks (other than shandy)

| | Almost every day | 5 or 6 days a week | 3 or 4 days a week | Once or twice a week | Once or twice a month | Once every couple of months | Once or twice a year | Not at all in past 12 months |
|---|---|---|---|---|---|---|---|---|
| Shandy (exclude bottles/cans) | 1 | 2 | 3 | 4 | 5 | 6 | 7 | 8 |
| Beer, lager, stout, cider | 1 | 2 | 3 | 4 | 5 | 6 | 7 | 8 |
| Spirits or liqueurs (e.g. gin, whisky, rum, brandy, vodka, advocaat) | 1 | 2 | 3 | 4 | 5 | 6 | 7 | 8 |
| Sherry or martini (including port, vermouth, cinzano, dubonnet) | 1 | 2 | 3 | 4 | 5 | 6 | 7 | 8 |
| Wine (inc. babycham, champagne) | 1 | 2 | 3 | | 5 | 6 | 7 | 8 |
| Any other alcoholic drinks? Yes .........1 No ..........2 | | | | | | | | |
| If yes, Specify name of drink . . . . . . . . . . | 1 | 2 | 3 | 4 | 5 | 6 | 7 | 8 |

Go to I7

54

O: N136/8 1oc'94 V2

I8. During the past year, how often did you have 12 or more **units** of alcoholic drink of any kind in a single day, that is any combination of beers, glasses of wine, or other alcoholic drinks?

This card will help you to work out the number of units.

[Show card 34 and use cards 35 and 36 as necessary]

| | |
|---|---|
| Almost every day | 1 |
| 5 - 6 days a week | 2 |
| 3 - 4 days a week | 3 |
| Once or twice a week | 4 |
| Once or twice a month | 5 |
| Once every couple of months | 6 |
| Once or twice a year | 7 |
| Not at all in the past 12 months | 8 |

(1–4) Go to page 2 of self completion, then complete front page

(5–8) → I9

I9. During the past year, how often did you have from 8 to 11 **units** of alcoholic drink of any kind in a single day, that is any combination of beers, glasses of wine, or other alcoholic drinks?

[Show card 34 and use cards 35 and 36 as necessary]

| | |
|---|---|
| Almost every day | 1 |
| 5 - 6 days a week | 2 |
| 3 - 4 days a week | 3 |
| Once or twice a week | 4 |
| Once or twice a month | 5 |
| Once every couple of months | 6 |
| Once or twice a year | 7 |
| Not at all in the past 12 months | 8 |

(1–4) Go to page 2 of self completion, then complete front page

(5–8) → I10

I10. During the past year, how often did you have from 5 to 7 **units** of alcoholic drink of any kind in a single day, (that is any combination of beers, glasses of wine, or other alcoholic drinks)?

[Show card 34 and use cards 35 and 36 as necessary]

| | |
|---|---|
| Almost every day | 1 |
| 5 - 6 days a week | 2 |
| 3 - 4 days a week | 3 |
| Once or twice a week | 4 |
| Once or twice a month | 5 |
| Once every couple of months | 6 |
| Once or twice a year | 7 |
| Not at all in the past 12 months | 8 |

(1–4) Go to page 2 of self completion, then complete front page

**D**

N1363        Self-Completion

IN CONFIDENCE

| Stick serial number label |
| --- |

Person

| | |
| --- | --- |

Date of interview

| | | 9 | 4 |
| --- | --- | --- | --- |

O - N1363D Jan '94 V3

1

96

PART A

Here is a list of some experiences that many people have reported in connection with drinking.

Please read each item and indicate if this has ever happened to you in the past 12 months.

If you do not drink alcohol at all please go to page 4

| | | Please ring 1 or 2 for each item | |
|---|---|:---:|:---:|
| | | Yes | No |
| 1. | I have skipped a number of regular meals while drinking | 1 | 2 |
| 2. | I have often had an alcoholic drink the first thing when I got up in the morning | 1 | 2 |
| 3. | I have had a strong drink in the morning to get over the effects of the previous night's drinking | 1 | 2 |
| 4. | I have woken up the next day not being able to remember some of the things I had done while drinking | 1 | 2 |
| 5. | My hands shook a lot after drinking | 1 | 2 |
| 6. | I need more alcohol than I used to, to get the same effect as before | 1 | 2 |
| 7. | Sometimes I have needed a drink so badly that I couldn't think of anything else | 1 | 2 |
| 8. | Sometimes I have woken up during the night or early morning sweating all over because of drinking | 1 | 2 |
| 9. | I have stayed drunk for several days at a time | 1 | 2 |
| 10. | Once I started drinking it was difficult for me to stop before I became completely drunk | 1 | 2 |
| 11. | I sometimes kept on drinking after I promised myself not to | 1 | 2 |
| 12. | I deliberately tried to cut down or stop drinking, but I was unable to do so | 1 | 2 |

2

3

PART B

Now I'd like to ask about your experience with drugs.
Here is a list of the most commonly used drugs.

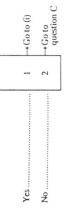

> 1. Sleeping Pills, Barbiturates, Sedatives, Downers, Seconal
>
> 2. Tranquillisers, Valium, Librium
>
> 3. Cannabis, Marijuana, Hash, Dope, Grass, Ganja, Kif
>
> 4. Amphetamines, Speed, Uppers, Stimulants, Qat
>
> 5. Cocaine, Coke, Crack
>
> 6. Heroin, Smack
>
> 7. Opiates other than heroin: Demerol, Morphine, Methadone, Darvon, Opium, DF118
>
> 8. Psychedelics, Hallucinogens: LSD, Mescaline, Acid, Peyote, Psylocybin (Magic) mushrooms
>
> 9. Ecstasy
>
> 0. Solvents, inhalants, glue, amyl nitrate

Please look at the above list and answer questions A, B and C

A   Have you ever used any of the drugs on the list more than was prescribed for you?

Yes ................ 1 → Go to (i)
No ................ 2 → Go to question B

(i) Which of these drugs have you used more than was prescribed for you?
Please circle the category/categories of drugs from the list in the box below.

1  2  3  4  5  6  7  8  9  0 → Go to question B

Now please answer question B on the opposite page.

4

---

B   Have you ever used any of the drugs on the list to get high?

Yes ................ 1 → Go to (i)
No ................ 2 → Go to question C

(i) Which of these drugs have you used to get high?
Please circle the category/categories of drugs from the list in the box below.

1  2  3  4  5  6  7  8  9  0 → Go to question C

C   Have you ever used any of the drugs on the list without a prescription?

Yes ................ 1 → Go to (i)
No ................ 2 → Go to D

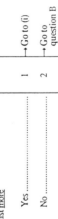

(i) Which of these drugs have you used without a prescription?
Please circle the category/categories of drugs from the list in the box below.

1  2  3  4  5  6  7  8  9  0 → Go to D

D   If you have answered 'yes' to any of questions A, B or C, please go to question 1 on the next page.

If you have answered 'no' to all of questions A, B and C, please hand this back to the interviewer.

5

> 1. Sleeping Pills, Barbiturates, Sedatives, Downers, Seconal
>
> 2. Tranquillisers, Valium, Librium
>
> 3. Cannabis, Marijuana, Hash, Dope, Grass, Ganja, Kif
>
> 4. Amphetamines, Speed, Uppers, Stimulants, Qat
>
> 5. Cocaine, Coke, Crack
>
> 6. Heroin, Smack
>
> 7. Opiates other than heroin: Demerol, Morphine, Methadone, Darvon, Opium, DF118
>
> 8. Psychedelics, Hallucinogens: LSD, Mescaline, Acid, Peyote, Psylocybin (Magic) mushrooms
>
> 9. Ecstasy
>
> 0. Solvents, inhalants, glue, amyl nitrate

**Please answer the following questions thinking about the drugs on this list which you have used without a prescription, to get high, or more than was prescribed for you.**

1. Have you ever used any of these drugs more than five times in your life?

   Yes .......... 1 → Go to (a)
   No .......... 2 → Go to Q4, page 8

   (a) What was it? (What are they?)
   Please circle category/categories of drugs from the list.

   1 2 3 4 5 6 7 8 9 0 → Go to (b)

   (b) In what year did you first use any of the drugs on this list?

   Please enter year → 19 [ ][ ] → Go to 2

2. Have you used any one of these drugs in the past 12 months?

   Yes .......... 1 → Go to (a)
   No .......... 2 → Go to Q4, page 8

   (a) What was it? (What were they?)
   Please circle category/categories of drugs from the list.

   1 2 3 4 5 6 7 8 9 0 → Go to Q3

3. Have you ever used any one of these drugs every day for two weeks or more in the past 12 months?

   Yes .......... 1 → Go to (a)
   No .......... 2 → Go to Q4

   (a) What was it? (What were they?)
   Please circle category/categories of drugs from the list.

   1 2 3 4 5 6 7 8 9 0 → Go to Q4

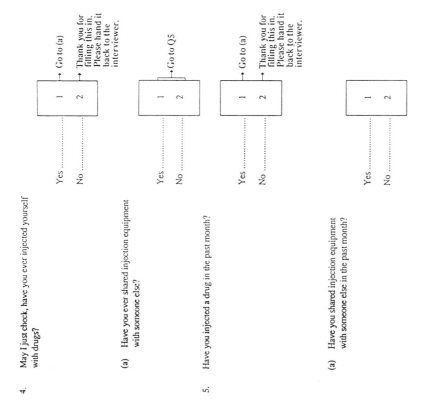

4. May I just check, have you ever injected yourself with drugs?

Yes .......... 1 → Go to (a)

No .......... 2 → Thank you for filling this in. Please hand it back to the interviewer.

(a) Have you ever shared injection equipment with someone else?

Yes .......... 1 → Go to Q5

No .......... 2

5. Have you injected a drug in the past month?

Yes .......... 1 → Go to (a)

No .......... 2 → Thank you for filling this in. Please hand it back to the interviewer.

(a) Have you shared injection equipment with someone else in the past month?

Yes .......... 1

No .......... 2

Thank you for filling this in.    Please hand it back to the interviewer.

OPCS, St Catherines House, 10 Kingsway, London WC2B 6JP

O. N3MD 1⚬94 V3

8

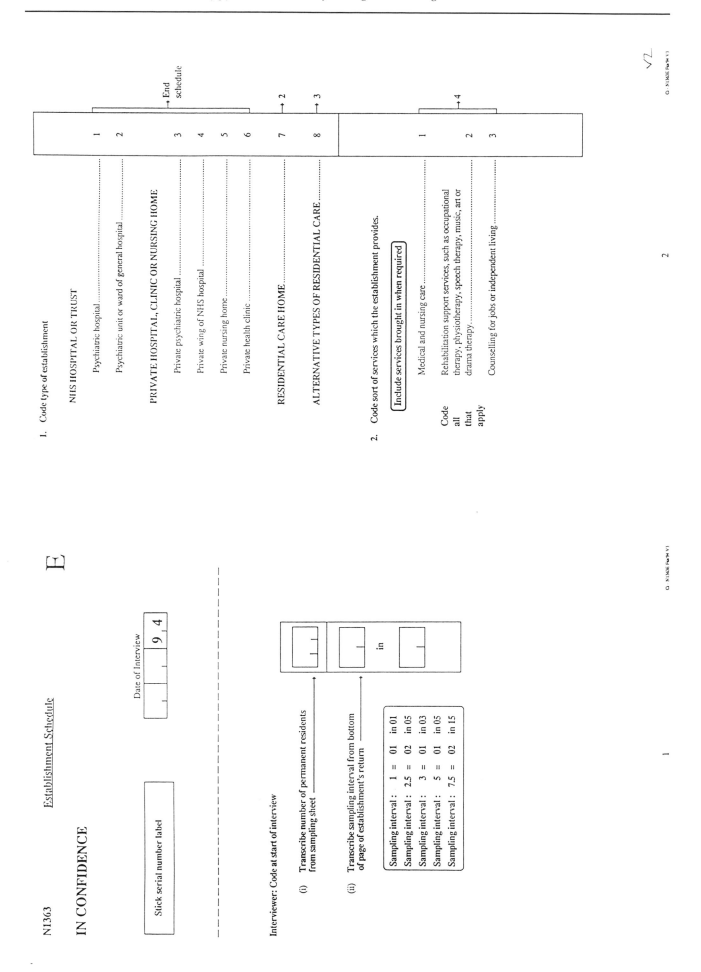

1. Code type of establishment

NHS HOSPITAL OR TRUST

Psychiatric hospital .......... 1

Psychiatric unit or ward of general hospital .......... 2 → End schedule

PRIVATE HOSPITAL, CLINIC OR NURSING HOME

Private psychiatric hospital .......... 3

Private wing of NHS hospital .......... 4

Private nursing home .......... 5

Private health clinic .......... 6

RESIDENTIAL CARE HOME .......... 7 → 2

ALTERNATIVE TYPES OF RESIDENTIAL CARE .......... 8 → 3

2. Code sort of services which the establishment provides.

Include services brought in when required

Code all that apply

Medical and nursing care .......... 1

Rehabilitation support services, such as occupational therapy, physiotherapy, speech therapy, music, art or drama therapy .......... 2

Counselling for jobs or independent living .......... 3 → 4

---

N1363      Establishment Schedule      E

IN CONFIDENCE

Date of Interview  9 4

Stick serial number label

Interviewer: Code at start of interview

(i) Transcribe number of permanent residents from sampling sheet

(ii) Transcribe sampling interval from bottom of page of establishment's return

[ ] in [ ]

| Sampling interval : | 1 | = | 01 | in 01 |
| Sampling interval : | 2.5 | = | 02 | in 05 |
| Sampling interval : | 3 | = | 01 | in 03 |
| Sampling interval : | 5 | = | 01 | in 05 |
| Sampling interval : | 7.5 | = | 02 | in 15 |

3. Code alternative type of residential care

**ORDINARY HOUSING OR RECOGNISED LODGING**

Unsupervised in ordinary housing with a degree of protection, eg from eviction if in rent arrears ... 01

Supervised ordinary housing with regular domiciliary supervision of personal care, household maintenance, hygiene, safety and rent payments ... 02

Recognised lodging where landlady has been selected for qualities of kindness and standard of care. Supervises personal care, hygiene, safety, rent payments ... 03

**GROUP HOMES**

Unsupervised group home where a group of people live together in ordinary house, protected rent, occasional visits ... 04

Supervised group home where a group of people are living together in an ordinary house but have regular (up to daily) visits by housekeeper for household maintenance. No care staff live in ... 05

Cluster of group homes where a warden lives nearby and makes regular domiciliary checks. Some built round quadrangle with entrance by warden's flat ... 06

**HOSTELS**

Supervised hostel. Care staff live in and on call at night. Provide regular domiciliary supervision ... 07

Higher supervision hostel. Care staff awake at night. (DHA) ... 08

Intensive supervision hospital-hostel. Higher staff levels than above. For people with severe behaviour disturbance or disability. (DHA) ... 09

SHELTERED COMMUNITY ... 10

OTHER (specify) ... 11

3

4. Code who manages or supports the establishment.

Code all that apply

DHA or Trust ... 01

Local Authority ... 02

Privately run ... 03

Voluntary and charitable organisation ... 04

Other (specify) ... 05

5. Interviewer check

If the address of your establishment came up on a PAF sample would you regard it as a private household or institution?

Private household ... 1

Institution ... 2

Not sure (Explain below) ... 3

4

Printed in the United Kingdom for HMSO.
Dd.0302175, C15, 2/96, 3397/5, 5673, 346403.

101